The New Ancestral Diet

The New Ancestral Diet

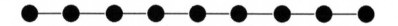

Richard Aiken MD PhD
with
Dagne Aiken

Go Ahead Publishing
2015

ISBN: 0692465715
ISBN-13: 9780692465714

Go Ahead Publishing
www.goaheadpublishing.com

To MARY BETH AIKEN

wife, mother, and editor, this book is dedicated

Acknowledgements

Creation of this book has been a joyful family affair. Many of the ideas presented here were discussed and debated in the Aiken household. Dashiell Aiken critiqued stylistic components. Quinton Aiken assisted with the website www.thenewancestraldiet.com. Richard Aiken and Dagne Aiken labored over content details. Mary Aiken edited every word.

Introduction

We as primates have struggled mightily during the past 85 million years to find and eat enough food for survival. Fortunately, every one of your ancestors was successful so that you might succeed in that same endeavor. However, today that survival is in jeopardy.

Recently and suddenly, from an evolutionary standpoint, the problem of subsistence in Western civilization has inverted: we have plenty of food but are not making selections that lead to long-term survival. Our plant-based whole-food ancestral diets for which we have become genetically adapted have become animal-based.

For thousands of millennia, primate nutrition *happened* while seeking *energy-dense* foods such as fruits. Today we still seek energy-dense foods, high in fat and sugar but in the form of processed foods and animal products. *Nutrient-dense* foods, formerly our staples, are rendered into side dishes.

Taste, the most primitive of our senses, over the eons existed for our survival (as all the other senses) to deselect plants sufficiently bitter as likely toxic or non-digestible. With the expansion of our brain capacity, taste was joined by higher brain regions' appreciation of *flavor*. The result is a demand for flavorful energy-dense foods. It seems that today *every* meal experience must "taste good" regardless of the nutrient content or health consequences.

This book is to suggest a return to our true ancestral dietary patterns, supplemented by what is known from modern scientific research concerning nutritional health. It is clear that we have evolved to be quite versatile eaters and while we *can* eat a variety of foods, a whole-food varied plant-based diet is best for our long-term survival as healthy and happy primates.

Following the high nutrient density to energy density ratio, we recommend a dietary emphasis on green vegetables, particularly leaves, followed by all colors of vegetables, beans/legumes, then underground storage organs followed by a modicum of grains, nuts, and seeds.

Personal opinions have been kept to a minimum. Most of the information presented herein is from recent peer reviewed scientific sources. For improved readability, these have been collected at the end of the book for each chapter section and subsection.

Richard Aiken welcomes feedback and productive interaction at his Twitter feed @rcaiken, websites www.moodforlife.com and www.thenewancestraldiet.com as well as Facebook pages Mood for Life and The New Ancestral Diet.

Eat like a primate.

Chapters

Chapter One

PLANTS AS ANIMALS

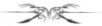

"Men as plants increase, cheerèd and checked even by the self-same sky, vaunt in their youthful sap, but at their height decrease".

William Shakespeare, Sonnet 15

You, and all your animal ancestors, have a close relationship with plants, and always have had, although perhaps not fully appreciated, as can happen in relationships – even vital ones. Although you may not have an emotional attachment to plants, your sustenance ultimately depends on them, so you do have quite a vital – even intimate - association.

In this chapter, these claims will become apparent as we trace the evolution of plants and animals. Given the vital dependence animals have on plants, the question arises: are plants subservient altruists?

Common origins

Let's start before the beginning. Earth formed about four and a half billion years ago from stardust settling, also formed the sun and other planets in our solar system. Collisions with other debris of primordial origin further contributed to the culmination of the fiery core of our planet, from which nuclear and geothermal energy originate.

As the earth mass cooled, steam was produced that created clouds in the early atmosphere from which continuous rainfall for thousands of years created about half of the water on our planet, the other half coming from collisions with icy comets. There were no recognizable life forms.

Now, let's fast-forward about a billion years, skipping the part where all the inorganic space stuff forms organic life. We don't know much about that process, although we do know that organic compounds, molecules that contain carbon and hydrogen as all life forms do, can form from inorganic reactants (witness the now famous "Miller-Urey" graduate student experiments). But growth and reproduction - creation of *living* matter – that's another matter. No one knows how life was first created.

You can pick your favorite creation theory - spontaneous generation à la Aristotle, extraterrestrial or extracelestial intervention, but the happy fact remains that *life happened*.

Supercell

Consider the very deepest root of our family tree with that simplest of ancestors, and our original one, the single cell *prokaryote* bacterium. There weren't many branches to that tree of life for some time. In fact, this superstar cell was the sole inhabitant on earth for about the next billion years. It remained present throughout the rest of terrestrial history and even to date as the predominant life form both in terms of total numbers and total biomass. The biochemical and genetic similarities between this and all subsequent living species, including you, confirms this as the common ancestor for all of life past and present. So as far as life forms go, we have always lived in the "Age of Bacteria". Even within our own bodies the number of bacterial cells outnumbers our own cells. Bacteria can survive almost everywhere on the planet, from the coldest to the hottest places on earth, to the bottom of the oceans, in radioactive waste, even on spacecraft. No other organism is as adaptable.

It's complicated

Finally, after their thousand millennial reign as the single earthly being on our modest sphere, about three billion years ago, these prokaryotes apparently further diversified into the more complex single-cell structures called *eukaryotes*, the common ancestor to present day plants and animals.

We say "apparently diversified" because the mechanism for that miraculous transformation is not known. There is, then, a very fundamental "missing link" in the evolution of the most important single distinction among organisms on earth even now: the prokaryotes and the eukaryotes. The prokaryotic cells may have provided an evolutionary substrate for eukaryotes, but interestingly they remained as a distinct simple cell structure throughout the succeeding history of evolution. There must be an overall advantage for the evolving earthly ecosystem to keep this diversity.

Perhaps it's a general rule in nature that the more diverse and interdependent the various species in an ecosystem, the more stable and survivable that system is as a whole. We have derived a mathematical proof of this principle for the simple widely used predator-prey ecological model elsewhere.

But not all relationships between species are as simple as the eater and the eaten. Consider *Rickettsia* bacteria.

Franken cells

On the one hand, the simple prokaryotic bacterium *Rickettsia prowazekii*, or *Typhus*, is responsible for precipitating some of the worst plagues ever to afflict the human race. On the other, recent genome sequencing has revealed that its evolutionary antecedent participated in one of the seminal events in the evolution of life as we know it. After it was "eaten" or otherwise introduced into the eukaryotic cell, the engulfed bacterium was able to keep much of its chemical composition and exist as a distinct entity inside the larger cell. This was a testament to the virulence of this particular bacterial strain. A new kind of mutual advantage occurred in this coexistence.

The new intracellular modified Typhus bacterium became known as the mitochondrion, the "cellular power plant" generating most of the cell's supply of chemical energy. So the "eaten" bacterium now within the larger cell is "fed" chemical substrates in trade for overall increased cellular energy, and the predator-prey distinction is obscured by this symbiosis. A Frankensteinien combination of cellular parts was brought alive by chemical "lightning".

The chemical processes taking place within the mitochondrion involve carbohydrates reacting with oxygen to produce water, carbon dioxide, and energy. This energy, in the form of a currency known as *ATP*, drives the growth, reproduction, and maintenance of the cell. Collectively, the many reactions involved in this energy production are called *glycolysis,* and although carbohydrates are the main fuel, fats and proteins can also participate directly, although less efficiently.

This aerobic respiration is why we breathe, obtaining oxygen, and why we eat, obtaining primarily carbohydrates and secondarily protein and fat as fuel for our engines.

This can be a hazardous enterprise though, because of intermediate energy carrying molecules, called *free radicals*. These free radicals aren't the peace-loving, anti-war protester types - they can freely cause radical cellular damage contributing to disease and aging. To the rescue come other intra-cellular characters called *antioxidants,* which we shall explore later.

Another perhaps even *more* profound example of cellular survival of mutually beneficial organisms happened about a billion years ago, give or take a few hundred million years. This also involved a bacterium that was taken up by a eukaryote - the *cyanobacterium*, also known as blue-green algae. That structure evolved into the *chloroplast*, a cell within the eukaryotic cell which provides photosynthetic production of energy from sunlight. Such single-cell eukaryotes evolved into multicellular precursors of present day plant life. Please refer to the illustration below.

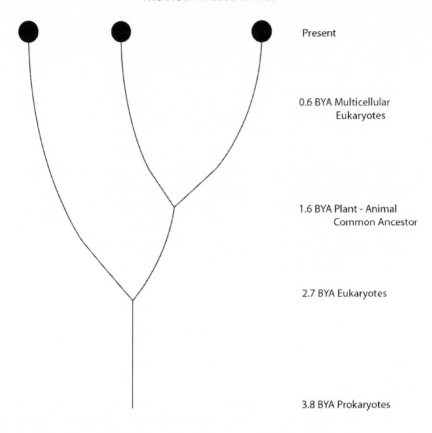

Present

0.6 BYA Multicellular
Eukaryotes

1.6 BYA Plant - Animal
Common Ancestor

2.7 BYA Eukaryotes

3.8 BYA Prokaryotes

Photosynthesis taking part in the eukaryotic cell marks the most recognized departure point in the evolution of plants versus animals, although the last common ancestor (LCA) was probably much before, at about 1.6 billion years ago. In the process of photosynthesis, atmospheric carbon dioxide, together with water and sunlight, produces oxygen and carbohydrates. This complements glycolysis (outlined above); so the plants provide the fuel (carbohydrates) and the fire (oxygen) for animal life.

This sun-supercharged eukaryotic ancestor of plants, however, is quite independent of the precursor photosynthesis-less coexisting eukaryotes which took a different evolutionary track to become animals. Plant life proliferated and as a result, the oxygen composition of the atmosphere increased to a level that encouraged the development of aerobic organisms such as animals.

Let's pause for a moment on that point. The aforementioned cyanobacteria, or blue-green algae, began producing carbohydrates and oxygen about 2.45 BYA that led to, after another billion-year buildup – dubbed the "boring billion" by some scientists – the debut of the first animals.

This is why animals are fundamentally linked to plants from an evolutionary standpoint. Our emergence as a species depended upon plants (single cells, then multicellular) and the continuation of all animal life continues to depend upon the existence of plants. Does *that* support the logic of a plant-based diet?

Common sense

All life has the fundamental biologic purpose to survive in order to reproduce. This life process ultimately requires energy and mass combining in an electrochemical reaction, a simple example being photosynthesis as discussed. Light energy becomes chemical energy.

This example reaction might be compared to a rudimentary process of food preparation, as all further use of the resulting foodstuff, here carbohydrates, is related to *eating*.

The obligate activity of acquiring sustenance and chemically processing it through eating is emphasized here in the beginning of our evolutionary timetable review, as it has always been and always shall be what everything else depends upon. Beyond all else as living entities, we must *eat*.

Intimately governing that universal eating process is that most primitive of senses – *taste*. One might immediately associate the word "taste" with an aesthetic judgment of the food source, but the primary point of this book is that taste, as all of the senses for all living creatures, has existed through our evolution only to assist our survival. *Food*, as a chemical substrate having the maximum nutrient value with the least expenditure of our energy, should be chosen and consumed.

Although there are tasty variations on the physicochemical mechanisms of single and multicellular organisms' food selection, the principle is remarkably similar in that a "probe" is extended from the hungry entity fishing for a nutrient source and, once identified as such through biochemical-structural means, is reeled into and through the cell wall for further scrutiny as the catch of the day.

Chapter Two expands on these utilitarian principles in the case of primate survival, while Chapter Five explains how recently taste and flavor have become a seductive source of destruction for Western civilization.

Plants land first

Land plants evolved on earth about 700 million years ago through a team effort by lichens and green algae in receding shallow pools of water.

The shift to land required some major modifications in plant evolution. This included the need for a substantial physical structure in the presence of gravity, a need less important when buoyant forces assist in an aquatic environment. This resulted in another major divergence of plant cellular evolution from animals - creation of the rigid cell wall.

This wall is made of cellulose, the most prevalent organic molecule on the planet. More than half of all terrestrial biomass is composed of cellulose. Even the physical book you may be reading is made primarily of cellulose.

The rigidity of the cell wall in plants led to a lack of mobility of the multicellular organism. Furthermore, the architecture required a high surface area to volume ratio in order to allow sunlight to enter the cell, again unfavorable for a motile species. This required the development of elaborate systems to ensure procurement of all chemical elements from a solitary and stationary planted position, and then sufficient manufacturing capability to produce all needed molecular components, including defense against mobile invaders. This demanded energy-intense chemical synthesis capabilities.

Fortunately for us all, plants have a rate of energy capture by photosynthesis that is enormous, currently more than 100 terawatts globally, which is about six times greater than the current power consumption of human civilization. Organic compounds are synthesized either directly using light as a source of energy, or indirectly through chemosynthesis. Plants also store some of the energy from light in the energetic chemical bonds within carbohydrate molecules that their mitochondria convert into an energy currency called *ATP* later at night, or at other times when the sun is not available.

Animal stampede

Eventually, as plants became well established on land, they significantly increased the atmospheric composition of oxygen (while reducing atmospheric carbon dioxide and cooling the earth). Subsequently, oxygen-breathing animals also evolved to survive on land. In fact, around 530 million years ago, there occurred a veritable explosion in the number of different animal species on land, called the *Cambrian Explosion.*

Rather quickly thereafter the morphologic diversity of animals was established and exceeded that of plants. This was because of the particular way in which their eukaryotic precursors aggregated and became multicellular organisms. It was the lack of a rigid cell wall that allowed animals to develop a greater variety of cell types, tissues, and organs. Specialized cells that formed nerves and muscles allowed mobility, a hallmark of animal life.

The motivation for this herbivorous animal migration to land, of course, was the plentiful supply of food from land plants. This again makes evident the evolutionary connection of plants as the natural food source for animals.

While animals have the advantage of mobility in their quest for plant food, plants possess the aforementioned advantage of highly flexible organic chemical synthesis. With the onslaught of attacking animals, primarily insects, plants used this manufacturing capability as a defense, producing so-called *secondary metabolites*, secondary in the sense that these substances are not directly involved in the growth and reproduction of the plant.

Therefore, it is a reasonable assumption that plants are not altruists. While animals might provide a convenience factor in, for example, pollination or dispersing seeds through their mobility and territorial placement of their seedy excrement, from an evolutionary standpoint, they are pesky intruders to be dealt with utilizing chemical warfare. Chapter Four chronicles this multifarious attack on all intruders, including animals and microorganisms; also the paradoxical advantages of savvy humans utilizing these substances.

Animals as plants

Both plants and animals have complex innate mechanisms for recognizing and responding to attack by pathogenic microorganisms such as certain bacteria, viruses, and fungi. There is considerable evidence that these basic and critical immune defenses have ancient origins from unicellular eukaryotes that predates the divergence of the plant and animal kingdoms. Perhaps even more remarkable, and alternatively, emerging data suggests that the analogous regulatory modules used in plant and animal innate immunity are instead a consequence of *convergent* evolution and reflect inherent constraints on how an innate immune system can be constructed.

In either case, the first-line defense of animals to invasion by microorganisms is quite similar to that of plants. This is important because of the potential myriad of bactericidal chemical components manufactured by our plant brothers and sisters could boost our own immune function. And they do.

Exactly how these plant immune signaling phytonutrients work in animals, humans in particular, is not generally understood, although the definite increase in our own *immunoglobulin* (abbreviated hereafter as Ig, a generalized antibody) production indicates that such plant compounds serve as a stimulating factor for human active immune response and is rather miraculous.

All nutrition originates from plants – all the carbohydrates, fats, proteins, vitamins, minerals one needs but there is an astonishingly vast number of additional advantages that plants provide through phytonutrients explored in later chapters.

To summarize, it appears that animal evolution was made possible by plant evolution. Specifically, plants were the universal source of the primary activity of animals: *eating*.

Chapter Two

Primal Primate Provisions

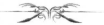

"It is not the strongest of the species that survive, nor the most intelligent, but the one most responsive to change."

Charles Darwin

The rise of the primates came with a varying reliance on plants for food – first indirectly through a diet largely of insects which fed on plants. As primates became larger, they based their diets more on fruits, then later shifted toward leafy plants.

This chapter spans more than 80 million years of primate dietary evolution. We shall indicate evolutionary adaptation from plant-based diets that led to primate DNA modifications which continue to date, *requiring* that primates include plant dietary sources.

Note that primate food sources during this time interval, approximately 97% of our primate ancestral existence, is devoid of eating other vertebrate animals.

Acquiring a taste

Taste is chemical sensation meant to recognize nutrients from non-nutrients. For primates, taste is determined by thousands of taste buds, each with hundreds of taste cells located in the lining of the tongue, the epithelium (see the following diagram). A protrusion of the taste cell membrane containing chemical sensors that interact with substances in contact with the tongue result in the sensation called *taste*.

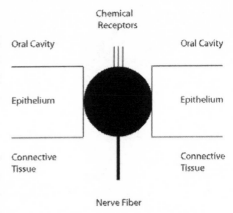

These chemical receptors signal the taste cell and cause certain cellular responses, including nerve impulses that travel to the brainstem, a primitive area of the brain, with the information that determines whether or not the substance is an acceptable food source. These chemical taste receptors are called G protein–coupled receptors (GPCRs), also known as seven-transmembrane receptors because they pass through the cell membrane seven times. Various types of GPCRs are involved in many other functions; for example, they are the targets of approximately 40% of all modern medicinal drugs. There have been at least seven Nobel prizes awarded for discoveries concerning aspects of G protein–mediated signaling.

Not being bitter

The most critical of taste sensations, developed early in our evolution as primates, was that of bitterness. Plant secondary compounds that have significant toxicity are typically very bitter. Detection thresholds for bitter taste are extremely low in primates, whereas those for sugars are also low but much higher than that of bitterness.

Taste receptors for bitterness (found in the so-called *Tas2r* gene) determine if the degree of bitterness is acceptable, indicating whether a given food is sufficiently nontoxic or to be avoided. This taste receptor gene set also is basic to whether a given species is an omnivore, herbivore, or carnivore. Herbivores have the most sophisticated set of these receptors, omnivores less so, and carnivores essentially reject any bitterness found in almost all plants.

The Tas2r genes in humans are thought to comprise about 25 different taste receptors, recognizing a wide variety of bitter-tasting compounds. It has been speculated recently that inclusion of more animal products into human diets may be limiting the full expression of this family of genes responsible for sensitivity to bitterness. On the other hand, olfactory receptor genes involved with sniffing out the environment have been inactivated at a much higher rate; over half of such human olfactory genes are nonfunctional. This likely indicates that dietary selection and general survival became increasingly non-olfactory during our evolution as primates.

This is why our primate ancestors likely favored ripe fruits when available, most having a low bitterness factor, but they accepted and consumed plants with bitterness under a certain threshold. That threshold may have varied depending upon the degree of hunger.

Many leaves contain toxic compounds, yet even among leaf-eating primates, there is a tendency to prefer immature leaves, which tend to be higher in protein and lower in fiber and toxins than mature leaves. The opposite is true of fruit; unripe fruit typically contains more toxic compounds and has a higher degree of bitterness compared to fully ripened fruit.

How sweet it is

The ability to taste sweet compounds evolved in parallel with the rise of plants bearing flowers and fleshy fruits. This taste sensitivity apparently evolved in connection with the digestive tract to encourage food choices that are energy dense and readily processed. This detection mechanism allowed an analysis of what might be perceived as edible or inedible, given the evolved digestive abilities of the time.

Primates developed a low taste threshold for sugars (i.e. high sensitivity), not only permitting the seeking of high caloric density foods, but also encouraging the utilization of a wide range of foods having a low sugar content yet perceived as edible.

Bitter sweet

Taste can be viewed from an evolutionary standpoint as the result of the need to estimate nutrient content and toxicity of potential foods. Taste operated in this way over the majority of primate evolutionary time, likely exclusively within only two spectrums: bitterness and sweetness. Other commonly identified discrete tastes of salty, sour, and savory do not appear to have had an influence on evolutionary genetic adaptation.

Arguments against the very existence of saltiness as a primary taste include no evidence of a genetic determination of taste sensitivity to sodium chloride or other ionic salts. The low sodium chloride content of natural primate foods is below detection threshold. The pleasant taste response of saltiness very unlikely is based on genetic adaptation.

Hence food availability as indicated by our sense of taste – sweet and bitter - strongly influenced our evolution: in a very real sense over these time scales, we became what we ate.

Primate time wheel

This chapter spans the primate lineage starting from 85 million years ago (*MYA*), with the emergence of the first primate, to 2.5 MYA, marking the beginning of the Stone Age or Paleolithic Period.

Consider this time period represented on a clock face with a full revolution being 85 million years rather than one hour. The accompanying figure indicates time intervals we shall study in this chapter.

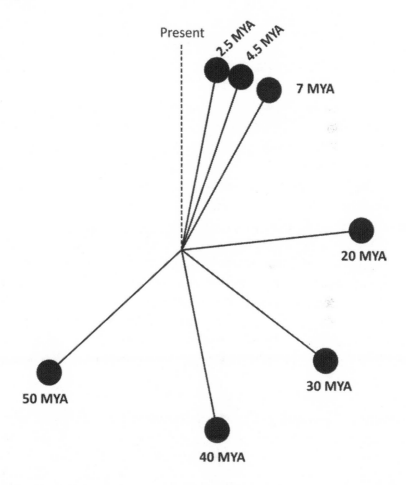

We will "turn back the hands of time" in each of the time intervals indicated in the figure.

85 MYA to 50 MYA

Rewinding to about 85 MYA, a type of mammal first classified as a *primate* diverged from the rest.

Primates are characterized by large brains relative to other mammals, as well as by an increased reliance on vision compared to smell, the dominant sensory system in most mammals.

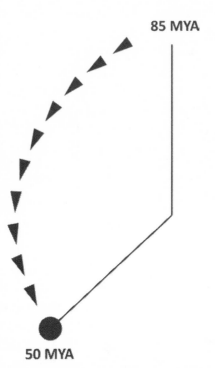

These earliest of primates resembled today's mouse lemurs, bush babies, and tarsiers, weighing in at 2 lbs. or less, and eating a largely insectivorous diet. Primate size appears to have had a significant influence on the nature of the diet; as primate size increased, many became more vegetarian, having diets of fruits, seeds, and leaves. An approximate cutoff point of 500 grams (about one pound) has been suggested as an upper limit for species subsisting mainly on insects and as a lower limit for those relying on leaves.

The obvious reasoning is that small insects are difficult to catch unless the predator is relatively small and quick, while the fibrous content of leaves and other plant parts require a more prolonged digestive process, and a small animal would be unable to maintain the necessary intestinal processing volume. Fruit, as a dietary component, suffers from neither of these constraints so was favored by a wider range of primate sizes. Wild fruit, likely more similar to that eaten by our frugivoric cousins, differs considerably from cultivated fruit in that it contains much more fiber, pectin, protein, and micronutrients, but is still easy to digest and metabolize because of its high levels of simple carbohydrates. The sweet taste is a gustatory signal for this highly favorable energy-dense plant.

One known early ancestor of all primates, called the *Plesiadapis,* had good stereoscopic vision with eyes on either side of the head. It was faster on the ground than on tree tops and began to spend more time on lower branches feeding on fruits and leaves rather than insects as was the common diet for other mammals.

Primate evolution accelerated with the extinction of the dinosaurs around 65 million years ago.

Berry berry

Our increased ancestral reliance on fruits and vegetables led to the loss of the ability to produce the essential nutrient thiamine, also known as vitamin B_1. Nobel laureate Linus Pauling championed the theory that after a relevant gene mutation, one or more of the animals living during that era must have lost the mechanism that allowed it to synthesize thiamine. This was advantageous to the animal – being primarily plant-eating – because it could obtain the thiamine it needed from the plants it ingested while conserving the energy it would have used to manufacture the vitamin.

With this energy advantage, the animal would flourish and perhaps have more offspring than others of its kind. The advantageous mutation would be passed on to descendants, who would in turn pass it on to their own offspring. Mutated advantages tend to become permanent adaptations.

However, with further unrelated dietary changes and adaptive mutations, there arose the dependence on inclusion of exogenous plant-based thiamine; otherwise several thiamine-deficient disease conditions could arise. The most common is a disease called beriberi that affects primarily the peripheral nervous system causing suffering through heart disease and paralysis, possibly leading to death.

Vitamin sea

A similar argument has been made for other essential mammalian nutrients that must be obtained through diet such as riboflavin, nicotinic acid, and vitamin A, supporting a very early reliance on plants as food sources.

About 63 MYA the "dry-nose" primates also lost the ability to produce ascorbic acid, vitamin C, first being unable to synthesize the terminal enzyme in its manufacture. This is yet another indicator that these early ancestral primates were quite dependent on a plant-based diet. All fruits and leafy vegetables are significant sources of vitamin C. By contrast, there are insignificant quantities of vitamin C available from animal food sources, except for small amounts stored in the liver. There are very few other animal sources of non-negligible amounts of vitamin C, lamb brains being one of the few exceptions.

Therefore, it was not only the norm for our particular lineage of primates to eat plants, it became a necessity in order to obtain this essential nutrient, unlike for most all other mammals.

Amounts of vitamin C required to avoid disease from insufficient dietary intake of this substance are likely very much lower than that required for optimal health. The exact amount of vitamin C required on a daily or regular basis to optimize health is widely disputed. This is a water-soluble substance that cannot be stored for very long in the body, so it is clear that substantial regular inclusion in the diet is indicated.

It has been suggested that loss of the vitamin C biosynthesis pathway, allowing rechanneling of energy and chemical substrates for alternative biosynthesis, may have played a role in rapid evolutionary changes, accelerating the emergence of human beings.

50 MYA to 40 MYA

The shift in diet of our primordial ancestor primates from mainly insectivorous to mostly frugivorous had been completed by this time interval. However, there was considerable variance among specific primate species.

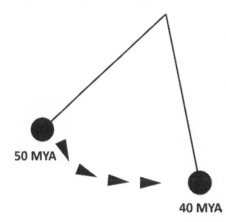

Fruiting plants by this time had replaced conifers as the dominant trees in the rainforest canopy. The feasting environment was the edible part of the canopy.

While ripe fruit offers high quality energy – relatively low in fibrous or non-nutritive substances – it must be supplemented with other food sources for protein, fat, and micronutrients.

As fruit and other plant parts became a more substantial portion of the diet, traits were selected that favored the processes of collecting, manipulating and eating plants, many of which became characteristic of primates. These included hands suitable for grasping, keen stereoscopic color vision, taste perception, and behavioral flexibility.

40 MYA to 30 MYA

By this time interval, primates were essentially herbivorous with little of the diet from insects.

It was likely that the flexibility and willingness to explore new potential sources of edible plants led to an adaptive advantage from visual and gustatory memory. Rather than just instinctual, this became an intellectual pursuit. Those food sources found to be of nutritional advantage were added to the primal primate menu. Scattered locations of a wide variety of preferred food were necessarily memorized and revisited as new growth offered replenishment of edible plants.

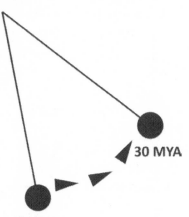

30 MYA

40 MYA

Exploration of new plant sources from the large variety available was likely a cautious pursuit. Possible elements of this experimentation might include the following:

1. Look for plentiful plants or those similar to known edible plants.
2. Choose the most plentiful part of the plant, usually the leaves.
3. Active evidence of parasites or a sour taste indicates rotting material to avoid.
4. Handle the plant so that it touches your skin; any redness or itching indicates potential toxins.
5. Place a small portion of the plant on your lips/ mouth and note any unpleasant sensation including extreme bitterness; if present, avoid the plant.

6. Eat a small portion of the plant and wait several hours; if there is any negative physical reaction such as nausea, do not eat any more of the plant.
7. With increasingly larger quantities of plant consumption, note if the plant is satiating and provides adequate energy. If so, continue usage.

Early primates necessarily became rather skilled with variations on these procedures. Aside from the universal edibility test, there may have been a few others principles regarding what kinds of plants to avoid or sample with great caution:

- Never eat plants with thorns.
- Careful of plants with shiny leaves.
- Careful of plants with umbrella-shaped flowers.
- Don't eat plants with white or yellow berries.
- If the plant's sap is milky or discolored, avoid.
- Stay away from plants with leaves in groups of three.

30 MYA to 20 MYA

Herbivorous diets became ever more varied during this interval.

The increasingly complex diversification of food sources and behavioral adaptations favored the development of increasingly powerful brain capacity, characteristic of advanced primates. Primate lineages that were particularly effective in adaptation to the environment prospered; those that did not became extinct.

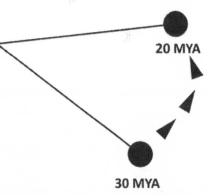

As mentioned previously, it appears that the core function of animal life was to survive long enough to procreate, and the primary activity throughout the functional life of each animal species was eating. While there were requirements concerning the dietary composition for each species, there had to be a consistent minimal intake of calories.

As calories could be so precious, they would need to be used efficiently. While the resting caloric requirements of the primate are fixed for a given species in time, adaptive evolution may select for certain variations. For example, the brain is an organ that places a rather high demand on readily available calories at rest. The gastrointestinal system can also require a high caloric demand to process food, particularly foods low in effective calories per unit mass as, for example, highly fibrous foods. The more intelligent primate can minimize the digestive/ intestinal caloric work by finding and consuming foods that are higher in caloric value.

Of course primates tend to have bigger brains than other mammals of their same general size, and this may have arisen from the tendency for primates to be more selective of what plants they ate – of even what parts of the plants they selected, for example immature leaves or low fibrous tips of leaves.

One particularly advanced dietary pattern may have been to vary the diet regardless of convenience by utilization of a number of local food sources. This is seen, for example, in present day eating patterns of the *howler monkey*, in which it is found that they do not satiate with a single preferred food source but will mix into their diet other fruits and leafy plants.

Primates may have developed dietary variety in part to minimize the potential deleterious effects of plant secondary compounds or to avoid over-consumption of a single plant species with a toxic component. The net effect, however, is a diet that more likely includes all needed nutrients and calories.

20 MYA to 7 MYA

About 20 million years ago primates lost the ability to make the carbohydrate called *alpha gal.* Other animals did not. We shall return to the important implications of this in later chapters, but merely note that it was in this time interval of our evolution that it occurred.

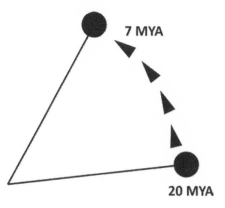

Dietary adaptations of ancestral primates now showed an even greater range, including hard-object food sources. Their non-animal source food spectrum exceeded even that of primates living today and especially the later pre-human primates. Their teeth were well suited for breaking down hard, brittle foods including nuts, and soft, tender foods such as flowers and buds; however, they were not well suited for breaking down tough plant foods such as stems and soft seed pods. This ability to eat both hard and soft foods, plus abrasive and nonabrasive foods, likely availed these early pre-human primates to be well suited for life in a variety of habitats, ranging from forest to open savanna.

These were the last common ancestors (LCA) of both humans and the modern ape family. Data suggest that the dietary shift in early *hominids* did not involve an increase in the consumption of tough foods; certainly there was not a preadaptation for eating meat. Here the term hominid refers to the group consisting of all modern and extinct Great Apes (humans, chimpanzees, and gorillas plus all their immediate ancestors).

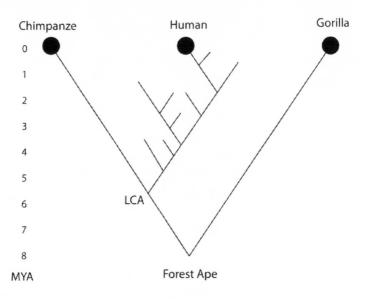

Chimpanze   Human   Gorilla

LCA

Forest Ape

MYA

The accompanying figure shows that there are three living species of African ape primates, and that humans are more closely related to chimpanzees than to gorillas. Human and chimp lineages diverged roughly 6 - 7 million years ago, indicated in the figure as LCA. This has been established mainly by recent DNA evidence and is quite surprising given that chimps and gorillas qualitatively seem to be more related to each other than chimps to humans.

Note also in the figure that there have been many variations along the human lineage that did not survive to the present; there were variations in body type and likely dietary patterns among them.

7 MYA to 4.5 MYA

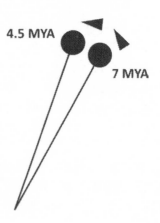

4.5 MYA

7 MYA

This time interval saw the emergence of the first known hominid (proto-human), the *root ape*. This earliest of hominid was at least a part-time biped that subsisted on a fairly generalized plant-based diet which included fruit, leaves, and probably

26

some nuts, seeds, and roots.

The brain capacity of these hominids was not appreciably larger than that of today's apes, so adaptive selection likely had not substantially favored an enlarged brain.

Fossil remains indicate that these creatures had massive molars well suited to a diet consisting of lots of tough plant material.

The environment was a dryish evergreen forest with no grassland.

4.5 MYA to 2.5 MYA

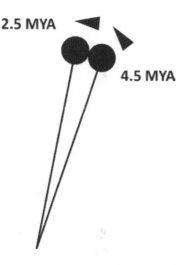

2.5 MYA

4.5 MYA

The dietary capabilities of these early hominids changed dramatically in the time interval between 4.5 million and 2.5 million years ago. Most of the evidence has come from five sources: analyses of tooth size, tooth shape, enamel structure, dental wear, and jaw biomechanics. Taken together, they suggest a shift to increased dietary flexibility in the face of climatic variability. Moreover, diet-related adaptations suggest that hard, abrasive foods such as seeds, nuts, and roots became increasingly important throughout this period, perhaps even as critical items in the diet.

Bipedal specializations are found in hominid fossils from about 4.2 - 3.9 million years ago. Possible reasons for the evolution of human bipedalism include freeing the hands for food gathering and carrying, changes from a jungle environment to more of a savanna that favored a more elevated eye-position, and reducing the amount of skin exposed to the sun.

By about 3.5 MYA, hominids in savanna environments expanded their diets to include foods derived from grasses and succulents common to tropical savannas and deserts.

Consumption of animal products has been proposed to have played an important role in human diet and evolution as forest resources became more scarce. More recently, it has been proposed that other dietary modifications and inclusions not of an animal derived nature, such as *underground storage organs* (USOs), might have been the keystone resources for these hominids.

No one knows exactly how frequently USOs were eaten by hominids, but it is likely that tubers, bulbs, and roots constituted a substantial percentage of their calories and became even more important than fruits for some species. In fact, one might speculate that a diet rich in USOs was so effective that it partly made possible their remarkable adaptive radiation. USOs are more starchy and energy rich than many wild fruits. They are rich sources of not just food but also water, and they tended to be available year round, including in dry seasons.

This accelerating development led to modern man in the Stone Age.

Adaptive dietary diversity

Let's summarize the substantial shifts in dietary patterns over the 82.5 million years spanned in this chapter. Roughly, primate diets changed from an emphasis on insects, to flowering plants, to green plants. Plant type was primarily leaves, but later included seeds, nuts, and roots.

In order to illustrate the range of these dietary changes, consider the accompanying figure, a so-called *right angle mixture triangle*

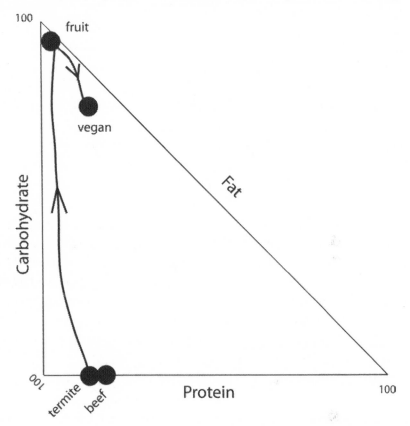

(RAM triangle) where percent caloric ratio for proteins appears along one axis and percent caloric ratio for carbohydrates along the other axis. Percent caloric ratio for fat is given by the distance from the hypotenuse of this right triangle, with values along that hypotenuse being 0% fat and values at the right angle 100% fat.

As stated earlier, 85 MYA very early primates had a significant caloric dependence on insects. The nutritional value of edible insects is highly variable, not least because of the wide variety of insect species. Even within the same group of edible insects, values may differ depending on the metamorphic stage of the insect. Our knowledge of the types of insects available for consumption back then and which of those were consumed is not known.

Like insects today, however, they probably consisted mainly of protein, fat, and fiber as well as vitamins and minerals. Specifically, present-day edible insects provide satisfactory amounts of energy and protein, meet amino acid requirements for humans, are high in monounsaturated and/or polyunsaturated fatty acids, and are rich in micronutrients such as copper, iron, magnesium, manganese, phosphorous, selenium, and zinc, as well as riboflavin, pantothenic acid, biotin, and other vitamins and minerals in varying quantities.

As an example, consider the present-day termite. On a percent caloric ratio basis, it provides 85% fat (primarily palmitic and oleic acid) and 15% protein. This point is represented on the RAM. Again, while there is considerable variation among insects in their relative percentages of fats and proteins, this is a rather representable value (grasshoppers are somewhat higher in fats – linoleic acid; caterpillars are lower in fat, etc.).

By contrast, meat – in the form of present-day raw beef, would be approximately 73% fat and 27% protein by caloric ratio and is also shown on the RAM. Both of these location points on the RAM – for termites and for beef – are very different from that area of the RAM representing the vast majority of primate history.

The shift from a diet more insectivorous to frugivorous occurred over an unknown time interval. However, this transition was aided by the relatively easy digestive processing of fruits, compared with other plant parts such as leaves.

Again, although we don't know the types of fruits that were available or chosen then, we shall consider common fruits available today to get some idea of the possible nutritional composition of the diet in those early days of the primate. An apple typically contains 95%, 3%, and 2% caloric ratio for carbohydrates, fats, and protein, respectively. Note this on the RAM; most fruit cluster near this point, being primarily carbohydrates, so that point is labeled "fruit".

It is at once noted the great variation in the relative location on the RAM of an insectivore (or carnivore for that matter) and frugivore.

The transition from a fruit-based plant diet to consumption of increasing quantities of leaves and other plant parts took a lot longer. Although the relative composition of which plants and which plant parts consumed during that transition isunknown, a comparison to the diet today of a whole-food plant-based vegan should give some rough idea. This is represented on the RAM, using 10% caloric ratio from fat, 15% protein, and from 75% carbohydrates.

Very roughly, the trajectory from insectivore to frugivore to herbivore is indicated. This illustrates the great diversity of dietary patterns throughout primate history.

Chapter Three

The Paleo Times

"Science is in trouble whenever the will to believe overwhelms the duty to doubt."

Siegfried Othmer

Our dietary patterns began to make rapid changes with the beginning of the Ice Age, which initiated global cooling between 2 and 3 million years ago. While the overall global trend was cooling, this did not result in a consistent local climate change in areas of Africa inhabited by our ancestors but instead offered more rapid variations in temperature, humidity, and rainfall. The overall effect with time was that jungles became interspersed and vast areas replaced by grassland savannas, woodlands, and other more arid, seasonal habitats.

Early humans evolved not to subsist on a single *Paleolithic Diet*, but to be flexible eaters, particularly so considering the changing landscape and climate, an insight that has important implications for what people today ought to eat in order to be healthy, as we shall explain in the final chapter on *The New Ancestral Diet*.

The Paleolithic Age (or Era or Period) is classically defined as beginning with the earliest use of stone tools (and thus corresponds to the beginning of the "Stone Age") about 2.5 MYA and extends to about 10,000 years ago (YA).

Hungry hominids

Hungry hominids had to be less selective in what they ate. This required increasing reliance on tough, hard foods such as stems, roots, seeds, and nuts. The result was an extraordinary amount of chewing.

As always, the most coveted food was that with high energy density, or caloric value, which did not require as much energy expenditure by the eater, including for acquisition, physical processing such as chewing, and for digestion. During this Paleolithic (Paleo) or Stone Age, many important advances were accomplished that made this possible.

While certainly hominids did not eat for fun and entertainment, taste continued to be a guide to identification of foods likely non-toxic, and to be energy dense. There must have been a certain degree of satisfaction when seeing or tasting a food source that was identified as safe and energy dense, but it is unlikely that "Paleo Man" relished the nuances of complex culinary preparations appearing in any "Paleo Cookbook" on the shelves today. He ate to survive.

As we shall see in this chapter, while food became more challenging to discover, advances in foraging and technical food processing met the challenge in full measure. In addition, more energy-dense foods allowed – or resulted in – profound changes in the hominid brain, contributing to the emergence of "modern man"- *Homo sapiens* - about 250,000 YA.

Stone: product release 1.0

While the jaw and teeth of these early hominids were adjusting to the challenge of ever more diverse food sources, another remarkable development occurred: *technology.*

Perhaps the first technical breakthrough consisted of finding stones suitable for smashing and later grinding of tough, hard food.   With limited manual dexterity, at first smashing or pulverizing the plant material was likely the extent of the "food processing" but later, as digital manipulation increased, grinding one smooth stone upon another became possible.

So imagine this scenario: a hominid is hungry, as usual. Hominid wanders along a body of water, perhaps a spring, searching for a familiar plant.   Once a candidate plant is spotted, hominid removes the entire plant from the ground, leaves, stem, and roots. Perhaps the root is washed off in the water. The entire plant may be chewable, but to assist this process a suitably shaped stone is found in the spring bed and the plant fragments - the leaves, stem, and roots - are pulverized into a form much more amenable to further chewing or simply swallowing as a bolus.

Certainly decreasing the residence time in the mouth by this external mechanical chewing assistance was not a taste compromise, as taste was a survival mechanism, not a culinary art.

The stone or stones that were used to process and consume the plant or groupings of plants were then discarded. This is a very important aspect of the process to note. The stone had only immediate value to the hominid. In addition to the likely problem of transporting stones, the concept of ownership was absent.

Of parenthetical note is the fact that this technological practice remains with us today in the form of mortar and pestle. There may be advantages in using this technique as opposed to high speed metal blenders that locally can heat up and decrease nutrient value through high shear force kinetic energy and cavitation (similar to boiling). Further, oxidation is increased from sucking oxygen into the highly exposed cellular contents of the blender as fibrous cell walls are broken down. But the point is that consumption of plant food is still assisted by devices that "chew" externally.

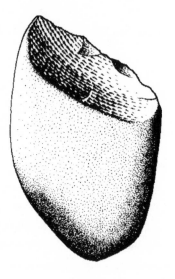

From about 2.5 million years ago with the beginning of the genus Homo, the first technical breakthrough occurred, defining the Stone Age of the Paleolithic Age: the creation of the first "manufactured" tool, the simple "chopping tool", illustrated here. It was created from a variety of stones struck by another stone causing a fracture. There was thus a blunt end and a sharper end. It was grasped by the blunt end, then brought down upon that which it was wished to detach or shatter.

Perhaps just as interesting as the emergence of this tool technology is the fact that this was the extent of hominid technological advances for a *million to a million and a half years*. That's about three-fifths of the entire span of Paleo prehistory.

Stone: version 2.0

It may have been that an advance in stone tool crafting was limited by our cognitive abilities and dexterity. The next technological advance was a creative leap about 1.5 million years ago: the *hand axe*. Here stones were flaked over on both sides to produce a sharp edge over most of the stone with a broad base on one end and a sharp point on the other. This required not only the identification of suitable stones for tool use, it required *tooling,* or processing of the raw material for more specific and effective uses.

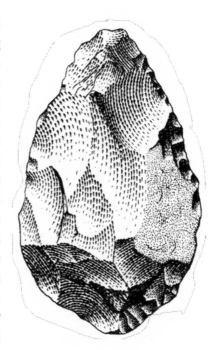

The earlier rounded stones remained in use after this new product release. In fact, it's uncertain exactly what the new technology was used for. Generally it functioned for chopping and scraping. It could have been used for food preparation, for example digging up roots, scraping off bark, or chopping down plants.

Markings have been found on bones of the era indicating that such hand axes may have been used to scrape off meat. Does this mean that these hominids were hunters and meat eaters? Unlikely.

Chewing raw meat would have been particularly difficult given the jaw structure and teeth of these ancestors (even today, chewing a raw brisket is difficult; ever give up chewing even a tough cooked steak?). There was no fire for cooking and breaking down protein cross-linked fibers to make it more consumable. Acid content of the stomach was likely insufficient to break down meat products for digestion, as were the necessary enzymes from the pancreas.

In addition, early humans must have been lousy hunters of other animals. They were slow and had no personal weaponry – no claws or teeth suitable for fighting. Very slow small animals like insects – termites, worms, caterpillars - likely had their place in the diet but certainly no larger meaty animals.

The hand axe was not a hunting tool.

Scavenging

An exception would be scavenging – waiting until an animal had died from attack by another animal or post-mortem from other causes – then taking what parts were edible. Some non-muscular internal organs such as liver and kidneys were possible candidates for the menu – if they were still available.

The timing of the scavenging would have to be soon after the kill, or the onset of spoilage would render the dead animal toxic. The distinctive smell of rotting animals is still one today that certainly must be primal and an indication of an unacceptable food source. Once decomposition begins, the bacteria, viruses, microbes, and other parasite populations inhabiting the carcass increase exponentially, rendering it not only indigestible but potentially lethal.

It may have been that after most of the meat and organs were scavenged by other animals, the bones remained, withholding their internal treasure until stone hand axes scraped off the rotting meat and the bones were smashed with stone tools for marrow. Bone marrow is almost 100% fat and thus a food source with maximal caloric density. The skull would hold a nice harvest of brain matter, consisting of mostly fat.

How often were these opportunistic scavenging events? Difficult to say but likely infrequent.

A feedback loop of increasingly complex foraging and scavenging, improving intelligence, and an expanding tool set began to spiral upward along the evolutionary ladder. There may have been the beginning of division of labor with tool makers, scavengers, and foragers, and the accompanying development of more complex social systems with a further selection for yet greater intelligence.

Out of Africa

The general drying trend included a component of unpredictability and periodicity, introducing seasonal cycles as well as irregular fluctuations in rainfall and temperature. These environmental changes led our ancestors along a trajectory to seek new food resources, including animal, as customary ones became less reliable and more scattered across the landscape.

However, it's clear that stone tools were not used for hunting but possibly for extraction and preparation of certain specialized animal products.

Perhaps a related phenomenon to this techno advance was the initial movement of hominids out of Africa about 1.5 million years ago. It is unclear why this migration happened but may have been related to searching for patches of nutrient-dense foods including animal carcasses. In any case, this migration did not appear to become well established. A migration of more intelligent progeny more than a million years later established advanced hominids over all land masses on the planet.

Advanced stone age products

Another *million years* passed before it was noted that the flakes struck from the core pieces making up the hand axes themselves could be used for specialized applications requiring varying degrees of size and sharpness. This takes us to about 250,000 years ago or the last *ten per cent* of the Paleo Age.

True stone projectile weapons did not appear until after 40,000 YA, or about the last 1.6% of the Paleo Age, indicating truely offensive hunting for animals. At last our ancestors, previously devoid of offensive hunting skills (even defensive maneuvers having been minimal), were able to attack – the only animal with the ability to attack from a distance, therefore compensating for physical mobility limitations, bypassing the need for close proximity to prey and lowering retaliation losses.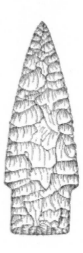

Mitochondrial Eve

Your family didn't slowly evolve in different parts of the world but came from one place in Africa about 200,000 years ago. And your original grandmother has been located; although we don't know her actual name, she has been renamed *Mitochondrial Eve*. Then, sometime between 180,000 and 90,000 years ago, a group of her progeny left their homeland, apparently with some advantage over every tribe of early humans they encountered who had moved out of Africa up to a million years prior. As they migrated, Eve's descendants replaced the locals, eventually settling the entire world.

The science behind these bold incredulous statements is exact – far more accurate than could result from examination of bony structures. Geneticists use mitochondrial DNA for tracing family trees because it's inherited only from the mother - not a mixture of both parents' genes, like nuclear DNA, so it preserves a family record that isn't scrambled every generation. Tissue samples from 147 donated newborn placentas from all over the world provided the data leading to these extraordinary claims.

It has also been found that present day human beings – from all continents – are a relatively new species. We are much more closely related than almost any other vertebrate or mammalian species. From a genetic standpoint, differences in human beings around the world are trivial.

Man fire food

At a place called Qesem Cave, modern man apparently gathered around a fire reusing the same spot many times by about 200,000 YA. Prior to this date and perhaps for hundreds of thousands of years, there was likely opportunistic use of fire for warmth, light, or ritual, but by about this time there are indications of controlled consistent use of fire. Although there is no clear archeological evidence for when cooking became common, it is the appearance of hearths, stone structures with an area for burning wood and an adjacent cooking surface that indicate the emergence of cooking around this time.

Of all the advantages offered by controlled use of fire, *this* was the most important: *cooking*.

Cooking increases the availability of nutrient calories in foods already included in the diet and expands the menu to include foods otherwise toxic or non-digestible if eaten raw. For example, tubers, including potatoes, turnips, yams, and rutabagas, characteristic of savanna woodlands and drier habitats, are very nutritionally dense yet almost indigestible raw. Harvard anthropologist Richard Wrangham and his colleagues have claimed that cooked tubers alone played a more important role than cooked meat in our ancestral dietary transitions.

Their hypothesis is that sexual alliances emerged from the adoption of cooking plant foods foraged and then processed by females, and that no other dietary plant had the same potency for promoting sexual bonds as cooked underground storage organs, with their high energy yield, predictable collecting locations, and increased value as a result of cooking. Apparently males wandering off hunting/ scavenging met with quite variable results.

Some anthropologists believe that hunting originally (and perhaps to this day) provided an opportunity for males to demonstrate their skill and fitness-related qualities as a potential mate or ally to the rest of the community.

Hunting requires a highly efficient and effective foraging strategic base, being a high-risk activity. Wrangham argues that meat was not an important source of food but rather hunting itself was considered an important behavior, less efficient than foraging for plants and thus possible only if supported by gains in efficiency such as provided by cooking plants. While that conclusion is not universally accepted, it is interesting that even today in Western societies, hunting is not an important source of food yet considered an important behavior by many, stereotypically by males.

Certainly it makes sense for larger primates such as those of direct human lineage to be *folivorous* (leaf eating) if such foods are abundant. Large bodied animals would struggle to meet their daily energy needs if they favored rare or highly dispersed foods, regardless of how energy rich they were, given that time and expended energy is an important additional constraint on energy intake.

As a contemporary comparison, the chimpanzee cooperative "monkey hunt" and subsequent sharing of food is a most dramatic example of meat-eating within the nonhuman primates. It is opportunistic rather than planned, and it has been suggested that chimpanzee hunting yields more social than nutritional benefits. For example, female chimpanzees are more likely to have sex with males who have shared meat with them than with those that have not.

Nor do modern human tropical hunter-gatherers rely on meat. For example, anthropologists James O'Connell and Kristen Hawkes of the University of Utah, Salt Lake City, found that although a hunter belonging to the Hadza tribe of Tanzania on average might catch one large animal per month, often weeks go by with no kills. The Hadza hunt with bows and arrows, technology far more advanced than that of early human hunters. Generally among modern tropical African hunter-gatherers, whole-food plants compose the majority of the diet.

Combining the results of archaeological and modern cultural studies, it was concluded that early "hunters" were most likely scavengers and male while the great majority of caloric value, dependable and regular, came from females foraging for plants such as yams, which would have been superabundant in the African landscape for millions of years.

Autoimmune disease and meat

N-Glycolylneuraminic acid (Neu5Gc) is a molecule produced by most mammals, but humans cannot synthesize it because of irreversible genetic mutations that occurred about 2.5 million years ago. It is speculated that this irreversible mutation occurred to survive a then prevailing malaria.

Neu5Gc is reported to be found concentrated in human cancers. As humans cannot produce this compound, the origin must be dietary – from mammals such as cows, pigs, and lamb. It is possible that the immune system recognizes Neu5Gc as foreign, and binding of anti-Neu5Gc antibodies may cause chronic inflammation. This supports the hypothesis that cancer is an autoimmune disease resulting in chronic inflammation.

Human ancestors dined on plants during the majority of the Paleolithic Age but did incorporate mammals into their diet toward the end of this time period. Thus Neu5Gc was introduced into the human diet, a *tumor promoter*.

Recall also that the ability of primates to self-manufacture the carbohydrate alpha-gal was lost about 20 million years ago. Other animals, many of which have been targets of the modern human diet, did not lose this ability and consumption of them introduces this compound into our bodies.

Bites from the lone star tick, which transfer this carbohydrate to the victim, have been implicated in the development of a delayed allergic response triggered by the consumption of mammalian meat products. Modern humans recognize the alpha-gal as a foreign body, thus producing antibodies to this invader. The anti-alpha-gal antibody is involved in a number of detrimental processes that may result in allergic, autoimmune, and autoimmune-like pathogeneses.

Dietary patterns in the Paleolithic Age

Very likely animals foods, other than insects, had no place in the actual diet of hominids for at least the first three-fifths of this time period. When it was introduced into the diet, it was an opportunistic supplement to plant foods and was likely limited to scavenging carcasses for bone marrow and brains and possibly organ meats such as liver and kidneys. The availability of such animal-origin foods was likely only sporadic but favorable for their energy density.

An ever increasing variety of plant foods was accepted into the hominid diet, including mature leaves, stems, roots, nuts, and seeds. These were the staples of the Paleolithic Age diet.

The addition of meat, i.e. animal muscle tissue, to the diet probably didn't happen in significant quantities until the advent of cooking, corresponding to the last 10% of the Paleo period. Even then, it was likely only a supplement to plant mainstays, which were also significantly expanded by the availability of heat processing. The preponderance of evidence supports the assertion that plant foods were predominant in the diets of hunter-gatherers.

The quality that best characterizes the actual diet of the Paleolithic era was *versatility*. Energy density was still the most sought after quality from food sources. Nutritional diversity, perhaps borne of necessity, was fed by the increasing expansion of acceptable foodstuffs.

Considering today's concept of taste, the Paleolithic diet was a "tasteless" diet but a survivable one.

Chapter Four

The Purpose Driven Plant

"And God said, Behold, I have given you every herb bearing seed, which is upon the face of all the earth, and every tree, in the which is the fruit of a tree yielding seed; to you it shall be for meat."

Genesis 1:29, King James Cambridge Edition

"Why should we plant, when there are so many mongongo nuts in the world?"

!Kung informant

Domestication of plants and animals produced an enormous shift in human nutrition and behavior. While this allowed for the development of civilization and further exploitation of plants for medicinal and industrial uses, there were nutritional compromises.

Agriculture originated independently in several parts of the world, with the best known early agricultural sites found in the Fertile Crescent in the Near East dating to around 10,000 YA.

The founder crops were einkorn and emmer wheat, barley, lentils, peas, flax, bitter vetch, chickpea, and possibly fava beans.

Emergence of grains and legumes

Certain wild cereals, or grasses, contain edible components in their grain, botanically a type of fruit. Many grains are a rich source of vitamins, minerals, carbohydrates, fats, minerals, oils, and protein and are energy dense.

The problem had been that first these grains must be separated from the inedible grasses, requiring some winnowing process. Secondly, the wild grains usually shatter when ripe, dispersing the seeds, making collection difficult. Then the tiny hard grains would have to be further processed to avail digestion. Thus, patches of such grains in the wild may not have been favored by hominids until at least primitive hand tools were used and present near sites of grain-containing grasses.

Sporadic wild grain stalks that through mutations tended to ripen without early shattering must have been selected patiently over time in early agricultural practices and replanted. However, this possibly led to other nutritional variants that may or may not have been favorable. Also the dietary patterns must have rather quickly favored this food source.

When the grains came

Grains and grain legumes were apparently consumed well before their domestication.

Compared to bone, plant remains preserve poorly resulting in sparse direct evidence of plants consumed in Paleolithic times. There are a few rare carbonized, mineralized, or waterlogged seeds and fruits, as examples, of miniscule groupings.

One such grouping, Ohalo II, was found on the shores of the Sea of Galilee. Dated at 23,000 YA, the site yielded a collection of ☐90,000 plant remains, of which nearly 19,000 were grass grains.

If the typical human generation was 20 years, that would place this use of grains at more than 1100 generations ago.

Evidence of starch grains from various wild plants was found on the surfaces of grinding tools at the sites of Bilancino II (Italy), Kostenki 16 (Russia), and Pavlov VI (Czech Republic). The three sites suggest that vegetal food processing, and possibly the production of flour, was a common practice, widespread across Europe from at least 30,000 YA. That would be 1500 generations ago.

Recent excavations in the Kebara Cave in Israel revealed charred remains of 3313 seeds, 78.8% belonging to the legume family. These were dated using electron spin resonance to be 48,000 – 65,000 YA. The oldest legumes found were from 3,250 generations ago.

Considerable amounts of starch granules also were found on the surfaces of Middle Stone Age stone tools from Mozambique, showing that early Homo sapiens relied on grass seeds starting at least 105,000 years ago, including those of sorghum grasses. This is more than 5000 generations ago.

Domestication of animals

Sheep, pigs, and cattle are species that were domesticated early, with the best estimates of sheep and pig domestication in the Near East being around 12,000 and 9000 YA respectively, with cattle following at about 8000 YA. Of the more than a hundred possible large herbivores that could be selected for domestication, these likely were chosen as they were herd animals and relatively docile. In addition, they are not territorial and lack strong flight reflexes. They also breed easily in captivity, a feature not universal among animals.

While agriculture emerged as a partial solution to food source problems for humans in different parts of the world at quite similar times, infectious disease added new problems. Agriculture changed patterns of human organization, concentrating population densities. This process intensified the spread of pathogens present among humans at low intensity of infection prior to the emergence of agriculture, and increased the rate at which pathogens infecting animals might cross the species barrier into humans.

Vascular disease

Data from various lines of evidence – anatomic, physiologic, and paleontologic – support the view that the ancestral line of humans was strongly herbivorous; certainly animal flesh was absent. Cholesterol was absent from the diet but massive amounts of fiber were present, enhancing cholesterol elimination from the body via the gut.

Cholesterol in the right amount is essential for proper functioning of cell membranes, as a component of transport lipoproteins and for bile acid and steroid hormone synthesis. Therefore, we evolved mechanisms not only to synthesize necessary cholesterol but to hold on to it tightly.

The introduction of a diet consisting largely of animal products, containing the animals' cholesterol as well as their dietary substrates for cholesterol biosynthesis, and saturated and trans-fatty acids, resulted in vascular disease becoming the leading cause of death in Western society.

This is in marked contrast to carnivores: they evolved to eat animal flesh and cannot develop vascular disease from its consumption.

Genetic mutations

With the domestication of mammals, another new food source became available, animal milk and milk products.

Through the millennia, mammals were weaned from mother's milk and then lost the ability to manufacture lactase, an enzyme that helps change lactose from milk into glucose in their digestive systems. Without lactose, consumption of milk can lead to digestive difficulties such as nausea, cramping, bloating, diarrhea, and flatulence, so-called *lactose intolerance.*

Some human populations, however, have developed lactase persistence in which lactase production continues into adulthood. Research reveals intolerance is still more common globally than lactase persistence (about 75% intolerant), and that the variation is genetic. Lactase persistence is now thought to have been caused by recent natural selection favoring lactase-persistent individuals in cultures in which dairy products are available as a food source. Based on living populations, estimates for the time of appearance of this lactase persistence mutation are within the last 10,000 to 5,000 years and has accelerated in the past 1,000 to 3,000 years, a very recent incomplete genetic modification.

In this transition to lactase persistence there is likely a spectrum of toleration that can lead to partial or periodic intolerance with attendant symptoms of indigestion. So this is one example of a genetic mutation allowing for the consumption of an "unnatural" food source taking place over a short evolutionary interval illustrating the remarkable adaptive capability of the evolved human. Just how many generations are needed for adaptations to various foods remains a question.

The transition from foraging to farming allowed humans to produce several foods in abundance that were previously less abundant, including grains and USOs. It has been shown recently that the copy number of a gene encoding a starch-hydrolytic enzyme in farming populations has increased. This study illustrates that genetic adaptation to the new domestication dietary patterns has occurred in humans since the agricultural revolution.

Apolipoprotein E (ApoE) is a protein that is essential for the normal catabolism of triglyceride-rich lipoprotein constituents found in meat. ApoE has a number of alternative forms that can result in different traits; the three forms are called ApoE2, ApoE3 and ApoE4. The ApoE4 variant, apparently predominant in pre-modern hominids, is a known genetic risk factor for impaired lipid regulation leading to elevated cholesterol, triglycerides and poor modulation of inflammation and oxidative stress predisposing an individual to a range of abnormal conditions from vascular disease to Alzheimer's disease.

However, this is less true of the ApoE3 (and ApoE2) variant that is dominant today (80%); the emergence of this increased frequency of the protective form of ApoE can be traced to within the past 200,000 years, possibly much more recently than that. Is this a result of increased amounts of animal products in the diet which add exogenous cholesterol, triglycerides, and inflammatories to the body? Likely. If so, this is another example of a genetic adaptation that has taken place over a relatively short time interval.

Another genetic transition has to do with cooking. Apparently the ease with which foods are processed in cooking has led to a genetic transition in which the size of the jaw is decreasing, resulting in a crowding of the teeth. This may be a factor in the vestigial wisdom teeth.

In Chapter 2, we mentioned the genetic mutation of more than 50 MYA that led to the loss of the ability to produce the essential nutrient thiamine, vitamin B_1. In 1897, Christiaan Eijkman observed that when chickens were fed the native diet of white rice, they developed the symptoms of thiamine deficiency, or beriberi. When he fed the chickens unprocessed brown rice, they did not develop the disease. The reason is that the outer rice bran contains thiamine. Processing in this case brown to white rice removes this vital component. This is an example based on genetic reasons of how "processing" plants can lead to an unfavorable outcome and why whole-food plants are preferable.

The genetic mutations that occurred many millions of years ago that led to our inability to make thiamine as well as riboflavin, niacin, vitamin A, and vitamin C appear to be unaffected by the addition of animal products to the diet, indicating either an irreversible mutation or that the inclusion of animal products was to a predominantly plant-based diet, even in the hunter-gatherer time interval.

Why didn't hominids over the past 250,000 years develop protective mechanisms for diseases arising from the inclusion of meat in their diet? Two reasons are apparent. First, the amount of meat in the diet was small and, second, such diseases only become significant if the hominid lives at least into what we consider early middle age, certainly past the estimated life expectancy of that era of 25 years. Natural selection is based on reproductive age.

In short, there is no genetic evidence that we have evolved to favor the consumption of animal products. We can tolerate it but at the expense of longevity.

Infectious diseases

Smallpox, influenza, tuberculosis, malaria, bubonic plague, measles, and cholera are diseases that evolved from infecting farm animals. Measles, tuberculosis and smallpox came from cattle; influenza from pigs and ducks; and pertussis (whooping cough) from pigs and dogs. The close proximity in which humans lived to their animals enabled diseases to cross the species barrier. This remains a factor to date, resulting in, for example, the flu pandemics that periodically kill millions across the world.

Diet was perhaps generally poorer for those practicing domestication than that of the hunter-gatherers, and may have affected adult stature. Just before agriculture was becoming common, men averaged a height of 5 ft. 10 in. By 4000 BC, males were averaging 5 ft. 3 in. Not until more recent times did average height begin to increase, but it has still not reached hunter-gatherer levels.

Hygiene issues concerning farm animals and humans in fixed close proximity exacerbated the spread of infectious diseases.

Why the shift from hunter – gatherer to domestication?

It is generally accepted that hunter-gathers were able to subsist adequately, so why would they change to domesticate plants and animals even at the costs indicated above? There are many theories, none generally accepted.

One theory states that domestication allowed increased socialization. Another that control over plants and animals was consistent with an emerging egocentric philosophy that man had a superior role over other forms of life. Still other views hold that technology, including that associated with cooking, farming, and concentration of individuals into communities allowed for a division of labor and trade.

Domestication of plants

In South America, potatoes and peanuts were early domesticated crops. In the case of the potato, domestication required a remarkable transformation to reduce toxicity; this eventually led it to becoming one of the most eaten staple foods on the planet.

Plant components toxic to humans are widespread in nature. However, the human body has many detoxification mechanisms that allow most trace or relatively low amounts of toxins without deleterious consequences.

Even plant crops commonly consumed by humans can contain toxic components. Consider the esculent farinaceous tuber – your friendly potato.   Even the best Idahoan contains significant quantities of the toxins solanine and tomatine that defend the plants against attacks from dangerous organisms like fungi, bacteria, insects, and other animals. These natural pesticides are concentrated in the leaves, flower, and stem and just under the skin, particularly in green potatoes.

In humans, these poisons destroy cell membranes such as those lining the gastrointestinal tract, increasing intestinal permeability and possibly contributing to "leaky gut" with associated inflammation and autoimmune disorders.

One advantage to eating raw plants is that some inedible plants containing toxic compounds are deselected from the diet, although cooking often breaks down such chemical defenses. In the case of the wild potato, however, solanine and tomatine are unaffected by heat.

In the mountains of Peru, wild relatives of the llama lick clay before eating wild varieties of potatoes particularly toxic to them. The toxins are absorbed into the fine clay particles within the animals' stomachs and harmlessly pass through the digestive system. Mimicking this process, the Peruvian mountain dwellers learned to dunk wild potatoes in "fixings" made of clay and water. Even today, this practice continues as many varieties of potatoes are grown and harvested in the Andes. The International Potato Center in Peru has preserved almost 5,000 varieties.

Through remarkable selective breeding 7,000 – 10,000 YA, also in present-day Peru, a more edible, less toxic, larger tuber was cultivated. The invading Spaniards introduced this cultivated potato to Europe and by the 18th century, famines were nicely reduced and the standard of living significantly increased across all of Europe because of it. Today the potato is the fifth most important crop worldwide, after wheat, corn, rice, and sugar cane.

Pesticidal ideations

This domesticated variety of potato carried to Europe and disseminated elsewhere, however, had fewer inherent pesticidal properties than its natural counterpart. Moreover, a single variety was cultivated and reproduced, yielding clones with the same compromised genetic vulnerabilities to invasive organisms shared by vast acreages across Europe.

From 1845–1852 an infestation of the mold *P. infestans* in the potato crop caused one of the largest famines in European history; a million people in Ireland alone perished – that country still to this day has fewer people than prior to that famine.

Later, in the early 1860s, the *Colorado beetle* created another wave of havoc on the crop. This time a series of arsenic-containing compounds accidentally when emptying paint cans were found to be toxic to the beetles and thus began the first historic attack of artificial industrial pesticides – to assist the tubers from the fact that their own natural defenses had been compromised with cultivation. But the adaptation of the pests to the ad hoc industrial pesticides was so fast that yearly chemical modifications were necessary. A whole new class of pesticides, DDT, produced after World War II, lasted a full seven years before frequent chemical variations again became necessary.

Recently, pesticide use has been linked to neurologic disease and depression.

Modern farming: hasty tasty modifications

This theme of removal of plants' natural secondary component defenses to achieve some desirable property for human consumption, and then the subsequent need to provide an artificial substitute for what was removed has reoccurred many times since these "potato battles" began. This may be to increase crop productivity, as in the case of the potato introduction described above, or to increase profitability.

A purple potato native to Peru has 28 times more *anthocyanins*, an antioxidant and anti-inflammatory compound, than common russet potatoes.

Bitterness, associated with secondary metabolites and phytonutrients, has been deselected by hundreds of generations of farmers, as has fiber, while sweetness has been emphasized. It is likely that many if not all of the varieties of fruits and vegetables we eat today are far removed from the original versions.

Candy corn

This sweet-for-bitter trade is illustrated by the "evolution" of corn. The wild ancestor of corn is likely similar to *teosinte*, a form of wild Mexican grass with "ears" consisting of five to twelve hard bitter kernels. Through mutations selected by farmers over millennia, a more edible and harvestable crop became a staple in the Americas by the 15th century, so-called "Indian Corn". While this version is perhaps less nutritious than its ancestral origins, it nevertheless contains high concentrations of anthocyanins, unlike present-day marketed corn. Today Indian corn is still grown but primarily for fall decorations similar in effect to the main use of curly kale as garnish for meat products.

Further mutations offered softer, sweeter corn. Scientific methods of hybrid breeding led Noyes Darling in 1836 to produce a much sweeter all-white variety, and in 1959, a geneticist named John Laughnan produced a white corn variety ten times sweeter than that, approaching 40 percent sugar. Along the way, of course, more nutrients were lost; for example, even the yellow corn of today has 60 times the Vitamin A (beta-carotene) than sweet white corn.

Monocropping

Industrialized farming relies heavily on broadly adapted high-yield crops to the exclusion of varieties adapted to local conditions. Monocropping vast fields with the same genetically uniform seeds helps boost yield and profits. Yet high-yield varieties are also often genetically weaker crops that require expensive chemical fertilizers and toxic pesticides. Diluting genetic diversity of plants is risky business.

Consider this recent example.

Ethiopia's east central highlands were once fertile with varieties of plant life, but by the 1970s farmers were growing only a few crops exogenous to the region but planted for high-yield potential. A devastating drought-induced famine of Biblical proportions there in 1984 resulted in nearly eight million famine victims and more than one million people died. One may recall the monumental televised musical production *Live Aid* staged to assist victims of this famine; the concert organizer and promoter Bob Geldof, who at one point in the show on camera yelled out *"give us your f---ing money,"* was subsequently knighted by the British Empire at age 34 for his efforts.

Once it was understood that plants local to that region possessed a natural resistance to potentially devastating famine-producing conditions, plant geneticists such as Melaku Worede reintroduced seeds native to the area resulting today in a healthy spectrum of endogenous local plants likely to succeed for generations. This was also an indictment of the addictive reliance on special fertilizers and chemical pesticides. There was no adoubement of knighthood for Dr. Worede for those heroic efforts. His interventions helped to advance a general appreciation for the inherent evolutionary advantages of locally established crops and led to a movement of collecting and storing native plants and seeds, known as *landraces*, from across Ethiopia. In 1989 Worede initiated the *Seeds of Survival* program, a network of seed banks that save and redistribute the seeds of local farmers across many nations.

It's unclear if there has been an extinction of the wild varieties of farmed food, but certainly it is generally true that local varieties of farmed plants are being lost forever at an alarming rate. In the United States an estimated 90 percent of our historic fruit and vegetable varieties have vanished. Of the 7,000 apple varieties that were grown in the 1800s, fewer than a hundred remain. Experts estimate that we have lost more than half of the world's food varieties over the past century.

Chemical plants

We don't know the purpose of most phytochemicals in nature – either for the plant or for animals. However, it is highly likely that the plant does utilize in some important way each substance it manufactures; otherwise it would be wasting energy, a practice of which plants are generally incapable except as an experimental mutation. And by "purpose for animals" is meant some specific function other than providing hydrocarbon fuel.

Auxin

Other substances have value to the plant but no known value to animals; for example growth regulators like auxin, which causes curvature of roots toward light, stimulates the growth of roots, and inhibits the growth of lower branches of trees.

Too much of a good thing can be toxic even to the plant, such as auxin in large concentrations in the synthetically produced defoliant Agent Orange used extensively to clear jungles in Viet Nam.

Also auxins in higher concentrations can stimulate the production of ethylene, another ubiquitous plant hormone of no known nutrient value to humans. Excess ethylene can inhibit elongation growth, causing leaves to fall, possibly killing the plant.

Ethylene

Ethylene is produced from essentially all parts of higher plants, including leaves, stems, roots, flowers, fruits, tubers, and seeds. It acts to signal a trigger for a wide variety of plant activities, such as stimulating or regulating the ripening of fruit, the opening of flowers, and the shedding of leaves.

A remarkable illustration of the use of ethylene for inter-plant communication and in the defense against herbivores is provided by the fierce defense of the *acacia caffra tree* from the predator *kudu*, a gazelle of the South African savannah. As the kudu begins to feast on the foliage of the acacia, within minutes the leaves become astringent, as the production of the secondary metabolite tannin is dramatically increased. Tannin, one of the oldest secondary metabolites known, has a characteristic bitter taste that the kudu knows is associated with low nutrient value as it inhibits the digestibility of the nutrients that are present.

Perhaps even more remarkable, the injury caused by the grazing kudu releases ethylene gas that travels with the wind to neighboring acacia trees and they similarly change from edible to non-edible. As tannin and ethylene production requires metabolic energy and resource expenditure by the tree, these processes cease when the threat is removed.

While ethylene has no nutrient value to humans, it is of value to us in other ways. It has been known for centuries that certain ripe fruit can signal other fruit to accelerate the ripening process. Apples and bananas emit particularly high concentrations of ethylene gas, so airtight storage of other fruit with them assists ripening. Industrially manufactured ethylene is used on a large scale for the same ripening acceleration.

Industrial ethylene production – hundreds of millions of tons of it per year exceeding that of any other manufactured organic compound in the world - is used as a simple organic molecule substrate in the synthesis of many other materials, including plastics.

Plants that existed hundreds of millions of years ago still provide the basis of energy production for civilization today through fossil fuels: petroleum and natural gas from aquatic plants; coal and methane from terrestrial plants.

Nutraceutics

Plants provide far more than energy and chemical substrates for biosynthesis – they can ease human suffering, promote health and vitality, and protect against illness – even helping to reverse certain illnesses. Typical such leafy plants are termed *herbs;* and nuts, seeds, berries, bark, roots *spices.* Throughout history, plants have provided the majority of treatments for disease and suffering of human beings. In the United States, at least half of the pharmaceutics approved for use in the past 30 years by the FDA are derived from plants. The pharmaceutical industry in the world trades about $300 billion annually.

Wise medicine man

Hippocrates, considered by some to be the father of Western medicine, allegedly stated:

"Let food be thy medicine and medicine thy food."

He separated the discipline of medicine from religion, arguing that disease was not a punishment inflicted by the gods but rather the product of environmental factors, diet, and lifestyle. The therapeutic approach was based on "the healing power of nature" (*vis medicatrix naturae*). According to this doctrine, the body contains within itself the power to rebalance and heal.

Garlic

Hippocrates prescribed garlic for a variety of conditions including for pulmonary complaints as a cleansing agent and for abdominal growths. Garlic was given to the original Olympic athletes in Greece as perhaps one of the earliest "performance enhancing" agents.

Because garlic was one of the earliest documented examples of plants employed for treatment of disease and maintenance of health independently around the world, including in Egypt, Greece, Rome, China, and India, we shall choose it to illustrate the use of food as medicine.

The earliest known references indicate that garlic formed part of the daily diet of many Egyptians. It was fed particularly to the working class involved in heavy labor, as in the building of the pyramids, with the thought that it maintained and increased strength, but garlic remnants were even found in King Tutankhamen's tomb, possibly left by a worker. The authoritative medical text of the era was the *Codex Ebers*, which suggested garlic for the treatment of a variety of abnormal medical conditions including abnormal growths.

This mention again of abnormal growths is possibly referring to malignancies of one kind or another, and it is interesting to note that of all plants studied to date, recent research suggests that garlic and other vegetables of the allium family, like onions and leeks, may be most adept at blocking human cancer cell growth.

In India, three ancient medical traditions, i.e., Tibbi, Unani and Ayurvedic, made extensive use of garlic as a central part of the healing efficacy of plants. The leading surviving medical text, *Charaka-Samhita*, recommended garlic for the treatment of heart disease and arthritis 2000 years ago.

A popular religious text of the Middle Ages was the *Hortulus Animae* manuscript which described plants growing in one cloister that were thought to have medicinal properties, garlic being prominently featured. A leading physician during the latter part of the 12th century, the Abbess of Rupertsberg, St. Hildegard von Bingen, focused on garlic in her medical writing. She came to the conclusion that raw garlic had more health benefits than cooked garlic, a point of view verified more recently.

The empirical observational skills of individuals of past millennia must have been rather good to recognize the health benefits of plants beyond the obvious value of caloric sustenance. The therapeutic efficacy of garlic does in fact encompass a wide variety of ailments, including cardiovascular, cancer, hepatic, and microbial infections, to name but a few. The elucidation of its mechanism for therapeutic action has proved elusive and a unifying theory has yet to emerge. This knowledge is limited more by funding than scientific capability as funding for nutritional research lags well beyond that for more financially profitable areas.

Today, at just 4 calories per clove, garlic is a nutrient-dense immunity-boosting superstar. One clove contains 5 mg calcium, 12 mg potassium, and more than 100 sulfuric compounds -- powerful enough to kill bacteria and reduce infection (it was used to prevent gangrene in both world wars). Raw garlic, not cooked or dried, is most beneficial for health, since heat and water inactivate sulfur enzymes and diminish garlic's antibiotic effects.

Food as medicine before written history

Physical evidence of herbal remedies from about 60,000 years ago was found in a burial site at Shanidar Cave, Iraq, where seven Neanderthals bearing a variety of serious wounds were uncovered in 1960. One of them was apparently buried with eight species of plants, seven of which are still used for medicinal purposes today.

One of those plants was yarrow, a powerful *healing herb* used topically for wounds, cuts, and abrasions, also known as *soldier's woundwort*. The leaves encourage clotting and reduce pain. Yarrow is also consumed as a mildly bitter leafy vegetable, particularly popular as a vegetable in 17th century Europe.

A common approach taken in medicine is to discover compounds in plants that have an important bioactive property in human health, extract and isolate it, and then market it for consumption in increased doses. Examples follow.

Psychiatry's founding fodder

The search for a mental state of perfect tranquility – without mental confusion or lack of focus – is a very human quest. In the tropical areas of the Orient, one substance was said to produce contentment without cloudiness, contained in a red-blossomed plant, about eighteen inches high, whose roots zigzagged along the ground like snakes: the *snakeroot* plant.

This plant was unknown to the Western world until the 17th century when it was described by a French botanist and dubbed *Rauwolfa serpentina* after the German physician Leonard Rauwolfa, who had explored the medicinal plants of the Orient in 1573. It was not until 1931 that five alkaloids were isolated from the plant, all of the phenothiazine family.

In 1951 Henri Laborit, a surgeon in the French Navy, was experimenting with antihistamines of the phenothiazine family to reduce shock in patients undergoing surgery in the military. He obtained a sample of a phenothiazine compound from the chemical company Rhône-Poulenc named 4560 RP, later chlorpromazine. Laborit did not find the effect he sought but did note a curious *désintéressement* (disinterest) present in the patients receiving the drug.

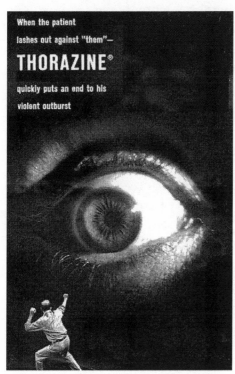

When the patient

lashes out against "them"—

THORAZINE®

quickly puts an end to his

violent outburst

Loborit, over lunch at the Val-de-Grâce Hospital canteen, persuaded three rather unenthusiastic psychiatrists to give 4560 RP to their patients. In February of 1952, Loborit reported to the medical press his surgical work with this substance, with a mere mention at the end of the article:

"these findings allow one to anticipate certain indications for the use of this compound in psychiatry ... "

A number of increasingly large-scale trials followed until by May 1953:

"the atmosphere in the disturbed wards of mental hospitals in Paris was transformed: straightjackets, psychohydraulic packs and noise were things of the past."

Thus began the psychopharmacologic revolution in psychiatry with the production of the commercial name for chlorpromazine - Thorazine (Smith Kline).

The first antidepressant, imipramine, was introduced in the late 1950s as an off-shoot of the tricyclic chemical structure of chlorpromazine. Many other psychoactive drugs are based on this basic structure.

Take two

Perhaps the first plant nutraceutic modified slightly to become a large commercial success was *salicylic acid,* found in particularly high amounts in the inner lining of white willow tree bark and central to defense mechanisms in plants against pathogenic attack and environmental stress. It is the principal metabolite of the medication *aspirin,* which works through a completely different pathway in humans to affect an anti-inflammatory and antipyretic response. However, dosing in isolated concentrated form resulted in severe gastrointestinal distress, so that a buffered form was developed – and patented – in 1900 as Aspirin (acetylsalicylic acid) by Bayer. This approach to acquiring medicinal benefits from salicylic acid is still flawed by the fact that there is an increased risk of bleeding even in low-dose therapy. About one in ten people on chronic low-dose aspirin develop stomach or intestinal ulcers, which can perforate the gut and cause life-threatening bleeding.

There is a better way to take advantage of the healing properties of salicylic acid: by eating plants. All plants contain salicylic acid and vegetarians have as much in their blood as omnivores who take aspirin supplements - but without the risks. Apparently this has been known empirically since the third millennium BC.

This is another recurring theme: plant-based diets can obviate the need for many supplements and prescribed medications. Plant-based diets are anti-inflammatory not only because of salicylic acid but because of their many other anti-inflammatory phytonutrients that help prevent the body from overproducing inflammatory compounds. Of course plant-based diets minimize one's intake of the inflammatory precursors present in meat and dairy products in the first place. More on that later.

Just to review, this amazing substance, salicylic acid, the active metabolite of aspirin and a plant hormone, plays a central role in the immune system of plants by activating the production of pathogen-fighting proteins. It can transmit the distress signal throughout the plant and even to neighboring plants. But the amazing fact is its crossover and apparent *inverse* role in humans: it *reduces* the immune response, i.e. serves as an anti-inflammatory. This has an important role then in chronic inflammatory states such as cardio- and cerebrovascular disease, stroke, arthritis, even certain cancers. Recently, mental disorders have been linked to chronic inflammatory states and aspirin is finding a use for disorders ranging from mood disorders to schizophrenia.

So this remarkable agent helps prevent disease in both plants and animals but by completely different mechanisms.

Chapter Five

The Science, Art, and Psychology of Eating

"The illiterate of the 21st century will not be those who cannot read and write, but those who cannot learn, unlearn, and relearn".

Alvin Toffler

After we had begun to understand the extent to which human health and happiness could be enhanced by a whole-food plant-based diet, the question arose as to why. Are plants altruistic servants of human health? I have posed this question to a number of prominent whole-food plant-based experts. Their responses have ranged from theological to simply experiential.

Our own conclusions are based on evolution. As explained in Chapter One, although plants and animals have common origins, they split into two quite different directions: animals focused on cellular diversity and plants focused on chemical manufacturing diversity.

The cellular specialization of animals led to mobility, but they were dependent on plants' abilities to grow nutrients from the earth and sun. Mobility also became useful defensively as some other animals eventually adapted to a diet of herbivorous animals.

But what about the defense mechanisms of plants? Again, the powerful chemical engineering capabilities of plants come to the rescue.

Members of every class of pathogen that infects humans - bacteria, fungi, viruses, worms, and insects - also infect plants. There are many potential invaders, so plants produce an enormous number of compounds that are toxic, repellent, or antinutritive for herbivores of all types.

Fortunately for humans, these plant defensive secondary metabolites that evolved over hundreds of millions of years were directed at the primary plant pests, mainly insects, and not toward the relatively sparse and late-arriving primates. As a result, while certain of these metabolites are toxic to humans, they are typically present in too small quantities to be fatal, although if consumed in quantity can lead to considerable discomfort and provide minimal nutrient value.

On the other hand, ironically, from the vast inventory of phytochemicals available, some provide significant *advantages* for human consumption. While a portion of those phytochemicals – let's call them phytonutrients - provide analogous advantages to animals as they do to plants, most act as chemical substrates for completely different purposes than apparently intended for plant use.

Let's explore several types of phytonutrients including anti-inflammatories, antioxidants, and fiber. These secondary metabolites of plants, numbering in the hundreds of thousands, are apparently considered "secondary nutrients" in that they receive little attention compared to those nutrients that appear on food product labels. But listing them wouldn't be practical as the labels would have to be too large, or worse, too small for processed foods.

Anti-inflammatories

As mentioned in Chapter One, plants have an immune system that is nonspecific to each pathogen, quite similar to the animal innate immune system; there is no adaptive mechanism, no immunity through memory of specific pathogens. The innate immune system of plants was previously discussed as a necessity of their inability to move about evading invaders and their extraordinary ability to manufacture defensive organic chemicals. Because of this powerful production ability of plants, many hundreds of thousands of such compounds are made for protection from the large spectrum of potential attackers. Some act as simple toxins, others in much more complex ways.

These plant versus animal innate immune system stories have similar plots but completely different characters. One "plot twist" in the plant immune system story involves the use of pattern-recognition receptors to recognize microbes, utilizing a large number of manufactured "resistance" proteins. Those proteins are indeed a vast cast, reminiscent of a Cecil B. DeMille epic motion picture.

Unfortunately the various immunity players in plants, while they do have analogs in animals, do not appear to be directly useful to animals in their immune systems when eaten, although they may be. We just don't know yet.

First, let's be careful with our terms. *Inflammation* (from the Latin, *īnflammō*, "I ignite") is part of the complex biological response of tissues to perceived harmful stimuli, such as pathogens, damaged cells, or irritants. Inflammation is therefore intended to be part of the healing process. For example, an organism may be infected by an unwanted microorganism, and inflammation is one of the responses of the organism to that pathogen.

It is remarkable to think that apart from accidents and suicide, humans primarily die from inadequate workings of the immune system. On the one hand, we die of acute infections from the inadequate immune response to invading agents; this is the main cause of death in third-world countries. On the other hand, we also die of prolonged or chronic inflammation that might be thought of as an overactive immune response; this is the main cause of death in the Western world and includes vascular disease, stroke, and cancer.

Epidemiological data as well as human intervention studies suggest that dietary patterns that emphasize fruit and vegetables are strongly inversely proportional to inflammatory processes. Example anti-inflammatory bioactive "non-nutritive" compounds in plants include carotenoids and flavonoids.

There are over 600 known carotenoids having a variety of colors ranging from pale yellow through bright orange to deep red. They serve two key roles in plants: they absorb light energy for use in photosynthesis, and they protect chlorophyll from photodamage. There is an analogous function in humans as an antioxidant in addition to its role in anti-inflammation.

Flavonoids are also present in a wide variety of plants. They serve many functions from ultraviolet filtration to floral pigmentation to attract pollinator animals. Generally, they are plant hormones or chemical messengers that serve signaling functions, most of which are currently unknown to science. At one time, flavonoids were proposed as a class of vitamins, Vitamin P, but this was not generally adopted.

While plants are anti-inflammatory, what about meat? We know that a single meal high in animal fat can cause an elevation in inflammation within our bodies that peaks at about four hours. After a meal of animal products, we develop *endotoxemia*, a condition in which our bloodstream contains bacterial toxins known as *endotoxins*. So inflammation is produced from endotoxins in the bacteria from animal products.

Bacteria: The unseen majority

Although there is a definite – and critical – symbiosis between certain bacteria and plants as well as animals, we focus here on the micro zombie-like invasion of plants and animals. Of particular interest are the defensive strategies of plants and animals at the cellular and molecular level in response to offensive bacteria.

Gut check

How do the invading microorganisms get inside our bodies? One way is the skin, the largest organ in the body. The skin is a very effective barrier – until compromised by injury. Once injured, our innate immune system springs to action immediately in an attempt to confine and eradicate pathogens.

But another body part has vastly more area exposed to the outside world than the skin – the gastrointestinal tract, starting at the mouth and ending with the anus. Of course its exposure is limited to what we eat, but there is quite intimate contact with whatever that might be. Unlike the tough multicellular barrier of the skin, the gut offers one single-cell layer between the consumed outside world and our body's inside world - the epithelium. We met this vital cell layer in Chapter Two in the context of taste.

It seems logical that the bacteria causing endotoxemia and inflammation after a meal of animal products would originate in the microbiome of the gut, namely in the large intestines where our resident bacteria reside. This was the *leaky gut theory* of inflammation in which saturated fat causes our gut lining to become "leaky" and allow our own resident bacteria to move into our blood stream.

It turns out it's even more interesting than that. It is the bacteria present in *meat products and processed foods* that bring the endotoxins. And it doesn't matter if the bacteria is dead or alive – even subjected to high temperatures (as in cooking) or highly acidic environments (as in our stomachs), because it is the biochemical bacteria-derived endotoxins, not the bacteria itself, that cause the damage. Saturated fat, also present in animal products, has an important role in assisting the endotoxin transport through the gastrointestinal endothelium.

Plants boost immune function in humans but do not trigger the immune response. Animal products do.

The B_{12} issue

An argument often given against adoption of a whole-food plant-based diet is that it doesn't provide vitamin B_{12}. How can it be that primates could exist for most of the past 85 million years eating only fruits and vegetables if they could not get this essential nutrient?

Plants cannot produce vitamin B_{12} but neither can animals, or fungi for that matter. Only certain bacteria (plus *archaea,* now classified as a prokaryote distinct from bacteria) can produce it; we can't even synthesize this complex molecule in the laboratory. The soil bacteria called *Rhizobia* that fixes nitrogen after being taken in by plant root nodules make it. Herbivores get their B_{12} from eating the plants that contain those bacteria. Carnivores get their B_{12} by consuming herbivores. Once in the animal gut, the bacteria can apparently proliferate and the nutrient is manufactured in the large intestine.

Unfortunately, it isn't absorbed there as such absorption would have to occur in the small intestine. Therefore the abundant supply of this essential nutrient appears in animal feces, including that of insects. This makes its way onto the external surfaces of plants and into springs and streams carrying animal excrement.

In our more hygienic world of Western society, we take special measure to wash plant parts, removing the B_{12}. Similarly our water supplies are treated to remove bacteria. Pesticides, herbicides, and other chemicals used to treat our modern mass produced produce reduces the amount of this bacteria that can grow in our soils. So the fact that whole-food plant-based diets are devoid of B_{12} is not based on genetic mutations or a need to eat animal products but on good hygiene and bad farming practices.

A supplement for B_{12} is recommended for individuals on a whole-food plant-based diet.

Taming the fire – the purpose of antioxidants

Recall that the defining moment in the divergence of plant from animal evolution was the adaptation leading to photosynthesis. The resulting chemical flame, or oxidative capacity, far exceeded that of simple glycolysis, the other energy production mechanism of plants and the only one for animals. As was mentioned earlier the highly reactive – and potentially destructive - free radical chemical intermediates require antioxidants to control the process of glycolysis. This need for antioxidants is even greater during photosynthesis, where very highly reactive oxygen intermediates are produced.

As plants adapted to a terrestrial environment from marine life, they began producing non-marine antioxidants such as ascorbic acid (vitamin C) and polyphenols. The evolution of flowering plants between 50 and 200 million years ago resulted in the development of many antioxidants in the form of pigments, compounds that reflect certain wavelengths of sunlight, appearing as various colors. Absorption or reflection of sunlight, including that in the visible light spectrum, acts to control oxidative processes under conditions of high light intensity present on land compared to marine environments.

The development of various chronic and degenerative diseases, such as cancer, heart disease, and neuronal degeneration such as Alzheimer's and Parkinson's may be attributed, in part, to oxidative stress. Oxidative stress has also been implicated in the aging process. Although the human body has developed a number of systems to eliminate free radicals, such as reactive oxygen species from the body, it is not very efficient.

We therefore benefit from consuming plants, the champion antioxidant producers. Humans, for example, have apparently evolved with such a reliance on plants as the source of antioxidants that we saw earlier in this book the fact that we no longer produce one of the most important antioxidants, vitamin C, present in all plants but essentially unavailable from animal food sources.

The primary fuel for our bodies is glucose, a simple sugar packed with energy. But you have likely heard of the perils of consuming products containing high levels of simple sugars, for example corn syrup. The problem lies in oxidation of simple sugars that leads to the production of free radicals, a dangerous consequence as mentioned previously. This might appear as a paradox, the most basic of fuels producing bad by-products.

The solution is *synergy*. Consumption of extracts from foods, that is, not the whole food, can lead to problems. In the case of high sugar content foods, whole foods such as fruits are energy dense with sugars but also contain antioxidants. So although the sugars do lead to oxidation, there is no oxidative damage because of the accompanying antioxidants. Without sufficient intake of protective antioxidants, only found in plants, excessive intake of the typical energy-dense foods of Western societies can result in cellular dysfunction, disease, and death.

Dr. T. Colin Campbell, famed epidemiologist and co-author of *The China Study* and more recently co-author of *Whole: Rethinking the Science of Nutrition*, remarks:

> *"Most importantly, however, we need to understand that these chemicals (nutrients) work in a highly integrated, virtually symphonic manner to produce their health effect. Thus it is a matter of thinking about the collection of such chemicals in large groups of foods. I hold that we need to discard the traditional view of nutrition, based on the effects of single nutrients, and take seriously the symphonic nature of food chemicals working together. In effect, the 'whole' nutritional effect is greater than the sum of its parts."*

Food synergy

Less than one half of one percent of all money for medical research is spent on nutrition, largely because there are no patented, profitable drugs that result. Most research conducted takes the reductionist approach aimed at identifying the molecules involved in biological events and examining them in their purified form or in simple systems. While this approach is understandable to isolate specific cause and effect, it misses the contextual aspect. Primarily epidemiologic studies of dietary patterns have been utilized, but this reduces the understanding of particular beneficial specific food combinations.

During the first half of the 20th century, a period often referred to as the Golden Age of Nutrition, all of the vitamins known today were identified, and good nutrition was viewed in terms of avoiding deficiency diseases - the reductionist perspective. This encouraged a collective vitamin pill supplementation.

Linus Pauling created the field of *Orthomolecular Nutrition*, "pertaining to the right molecule". Pauling proposed that by giving the body the right molecules in the right concentration, nutrients could be used by people to achieve better health and prolong life. He advocated the popular but controversial *megavitamin therapy* movement of the 1970s, particularly for vitamin C. This was a natural reductionist approach for a Nobel Prize winning molecular chemist but is widely considered to be a medical fail.

The concept of food synergy is based instead on the idea that the interrelations between constituents in foods are significant. But this is also true between foods, that is combinations of different whole foods.

For example, the plant turmeric, containing the ingredient curcumin, appears to have a wide range of biological effects including anti-inflammatory, antioxidant, antibacterial, and antiviral, but is poorly absorbed, or has low *bioavailability*. With the addition of black pepper, and its active ingredient *piperine*, the bioavailability increases by 2000%.

The synergy likely works best with a variety of different fruits and vegetables. Extracts of phytonutrients, such as curcumin just mentioned, could have deleterious effects. As phytonutrients have medicinal properties, it's probably best not to flood one's diet with only a few plant sources.

There are specific examples of food combinations that appear to have synergy. Fats make carotenoids more bioavailable, so a combination of tomatoes and avocados may be a good combination. Tomatoes and broccoli both have anti-prostate tumor properties but the combination is better than the sum of the effects individually. Eating two different fruits together has a greater antioxidant capacity than the same amount of either fruit consumed individually. Vitamin C helps to make iron more absorbable so a combination of fruit with iron-containing vegetables (leeks, beet greens, kale, spinach, etc.) may be particularly effective for this purpose.

More bang for the bulk

Some animals that eat other animals are somewhat selective about what part of the carcass they consume. Most animals do not eat the bones of other animals, presumably because of mastication or digestive limitations.

While plants have no skeletal system per se, they do have a rigid enough structure to keep them upright. This is primarily a result of their rigid cell walls, discussed briefly earlier as an evolutionary choice a strain of eukaryotes happened to make. Technically, it's not just the rigidity of the cell wall, but the tensile strength of the wall combined with hydraulic pressure from within the cell that keeps it rigid. Observe a plant wilting from lack of water to illustrate.

The plant cell wall performs many functions besides structure and thus its chemical composition is somewhat complex; certainly the major constituent of the cell wall of green plants is cellulose, the most abundant organic polymer on earth.

It used to be, as we learned in high school, cellulose was equated with fiber, and fiber in the diet was primarily a consideration for regularity in bowel movement. There is much more to the story than that.

The definition of *fiber* is not consistently accepted. First fiber was defined to be the components of plants that resist human digestive enzymes, a definition that added to cellulose other material such as lignin, a "woody" organic polymer not quite as plentiful as cellulose. The next addition to the definition of fiber were certain water soluble materials that were easily fermented by gut bacteria and resulted in physiologically active prebiotic byproducts. A third addition was "resistant starch", those starches that resist digestion and absorption in the small intestine.

It would seem now that fiber is basically plant material that can change the gastrointestinal tract, including the microbiome by changing how other nutrients are absorbed. So fiber is far from inert substances that go along for the ride so you can go along to the bathroom.

While human enzymes may not be able to digest dietary fiber, it is digestible by our gut bacteria, which make short chain fatty acids from it, inhibiting the growth of harmful gut bacteria, increasing mineral absorption such as calcium, stimulating blood flow as well as colonic fluid and electrolyte uptake. Furthermore, there may be important digestible phytonutrients that are chemically attached to the fibrous content and released during processing by our micro flora.

There may be an additional evolutionary effect from millions of years of primates consuming significant amounts of fiber: satiation. Diets high in fiber do fill the stomach and reduce the drive to eat. A diet low in fiber but energy dense would lead to extra caloric consumption prior to satiation. If this becomes a consistent pattern, as in human diets currently in Western cultures, it contributes to obesity.

Food as art

Generally art is difficult to define but simply put it is the appreciated product of creative human play. Play in the sense of Mark Twain:

> *"Work consists of whatever a body is obliged to do. Play consists of whatever a body is not obliged to do."*

Using this definition, art is a relatively new hominid concept, at least at the level of current appreciation. Art relates first to the senses, then the emotions often by association. The sense of sound lends itself to music, vision to the visual arts, touch to tactile physical stimulation. A sentiment of some individuals in advanced societies is *the earth without art* is *"eh"*.

What about taste? Taste remains as the most primitive of senses with its basic function of survival. Eating has been our most important activity, besides procreating, and food source selection has been based for the most part on taste.

However, in current society we have identified safe food sources, very much reducing the critical function of taste for survival. We have previously explored the evolutionary adaptation of taste being divided into two types: bitter and sweet. These taste fibers are hardwired at the brainstem level. There have now been identified additional taste receptors for different nuances of taste that do not appear fundamental to our genetic makeup such as saltiness, sourness, and savoriness or umami.

These relatively recent additional taste sensations have a role in the artistic development of culinary art, but likely a minor one, compared to the advancement of smell. Primates have never had the sensitive sense of smell that many other animals have of their external environment, but there is another advanced different type of smell involved in human artistic appreciation of consumed food sources that surpasses that sense in all other animals: this smell is involved with the appreciation of flavor.

Neurogastronomy

There are two very different neurochemical pathways involved in human perception of smell: exterior or frontal smell, also called orthonasal smell, as in many other animals, and posterior or retronasal smell. This latter type of smell is much different from the former: it has receptor fibers for volatile gases that directly connect to the frontal cortex, a highly intellectual area of the brain. It is this retronasal smell, combined with taste, that leads to the artistic realm of flavor.

So if one judges a food to have a good taste, that person is actually making judgment on its *flavor*. This is an important finding. Tastes are rather fixed; most everyone has similar perception of sweet and bitter, for example, although there are varying sensitivities among individuals. However flavor, being an interpretive higher cognitive function, can be influenced by association.

Much of the brain is integrated. Neuronal fibers from the smell regions of the frontal cortex communicate with diverse areas of the brain having to do with memory, emotion, and behavior. There are also connections to various other areas of the prefrontal cortex involved in learning and decision making, so-called executive function. Even the way food looks (presentation) and feels in our mouth (texture) has some influence on the overall perception of flavor.

These advanced brain regions are not fully developed until well into adulthood, perhaps explaining the culinary reluctance and more limited dietary patterns of children and adolescents.

That flavor is highly influenced by retronasal smell is evident to anyone with a "stuffy nose". This can also be simulated by pinching the nose or by mouth breathing only. This does not affect the taste receptors so can be an interesting experiment to detect, for example, bitter and sweet taste thresholds without the influence of flavor.

The tasteless diet

Flavor can be a beautiful thing and is the basis for the culinary arts. But it shouldn't *always* be the basis of one's diet – that should still be survival, and that means selection of nutrient-dense foods in addition to some energy-dense foods.

Consider the analogous situation for the other senses. For example, we enjoy hearing beautiful music but usually use our sense of hearing for more practical purposes. Similarly, we may enjoy the visual arts but primarily use this sense in a utilitarian way to function safely.

To rethink one's flavor and taste associations, consider a cognitive behavioral approach.

Cognitive behavioral tasting: it's the thought that counts

The most effective and common therapeutic approach to controlling one's thinking, emotions, and behavior in the United States is a technique called Cognitive Behavioral Therapy (CBT). It is a model of the human experience in that a sensorial stimulation (visual, auditory, tactile, taste, or olfactory) provides the *trigger* for an *automatic thought* based on previous conditioning of that sensation. The automatic thought then is associated with an *emotion* that leads to a behavior or *response*. This is represented in the accompanying figure using the acronym TATER, where the letters stand for: T = Trigger; AT = automatic thought; E = emotion; and R = response.

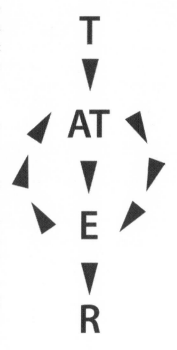

The idea in therapeutic use of CBT is to interrupt this sequence once an unpleasant emotion is encountered and rethink the automatic thought that resulted from the triggering sensation. This is shown in the TATER figure by the revolving arrows at the level of AT, the automatic thought. Successful challenge of the automatic thought using more positive rational thinking then can lead to an improved emotional outcome and therefore behavior.

This principle could be extended for use with flavor associations, similar to an "acquired taste". For example some highly nutritious foods are low in fat, salt, and sugars and may not be as palatable as some less nutritious energy-dense foods. Tasting such foods may first be met with a negative automatic thought but subsequent tastings, coupled with the knowledge of the positive nutrient effect on one's health, may lead to a more acceptable flavor association.

Furthermore, CBT principles can be used to develop and adhere to a healthy dietary pattern as it becomes part of one's natural lifestyle.

Fork in the road

In this chapter we have reviewed just some of the advantages that whole-food plant-based diets can have for human consumption, and we didn't even get into the macronutrients, vitamins, and minerals so plentiful in plants. We are only beginning to appreciate what plants bring to the table to assist our health and happiness.

Just to summarize, plants don't particularly like animals, nor do they have much need of them; generally, they would like to kill animals. However, in the case of the human animal, the great chemical manufacturing capability of plants has proven to be very beneficial even beyond our ultimate dependence on plants for basic energy needs.

Foods eaten by humans today, especially those consumed in industrialized nations, bear little resemblance to the plant-based diets anthropods have favored since their emergence. This lends support to the notion that many health problems common in technologically advanced nations may result in part from a mismatch between diets we now eat and those to which our bodies have become adapted over millions of years.

Within the evolutionary medicine literature, the origin of agriculture tends to be seen as the primary point at which dietary 'adaptation' switches to 'maladaptation' within humans.

Chapter Six

Mood Food

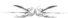

"You may be an undigested bit of beef, a blot of mustard, a crumb of cheese, a fragment of underdone potato. There's more of gravy than of grave about you, whatever you are!"

Charles Dickens, *A Christmas Carol*

Human emotion and behavior is governed by a most sensitive and nutrionally demanding organ – the brain. While the importance of diet on *cardio*-vascular health is emphasized in the literature, *neuro*-vascular health is equally important.

Adult dietary patterns and mood

Even though most medications used in psychiatry are derived directly from plant secondary metabolites or patented variations, only recently have psychiatrists begun to consider the healing power of plants themselves. The March 2010 issue of the so-called "green journal", the most prestigious and conservative journal of the American Psychiatric Association, actually featured dietary considerations as related to psychiatric disorders.

An editorial appeared in that issue, written by Marlene Freeman, M.D. and Associate Professor in the Department of Psychiatry at Harvard Medical School, in which she noted:

"It is both compelling and daunting that dietary interventions at an individual or population level could reduce rates of psychiatric disorders."

One study in that issue is titled "Association of Western and Traditional Diets With Depression and Anxiety in Women." In this and all research into the relationship between diet quality and emotional states, there is always the challenge of *defining* and *measuring* diet quality and mood. There is no accepted "gold standard" measure of either.

With that in mind, this was a study of about one thousand adult women who were examined over a short time interval, a so-called cross-sectional study. Their conclusion was that:

"a 'traditional' dietary pattern characterized by vegetables, fruit, meat, fish, and whole grains was associated with lower odds for major depression or dysthymia and for anxiety disorders. A 'Western' diet of processed or fried foods, refined grains, sugary products, and beer was associated with a higher GHQ-12 score."

The GHQ-12 is a measure of emotional health, a 12-item questionnaire asked of each participant – the lower the score the better. More generally, the authors state:

"There was also an inverse association between diet quality score and GHQ-12 score".

Again "diet quality" was defined by a particular food frequency questionnaire utilized, so by their definitions, a better diet quality resulted in better emotional states. By their measures, a "Western Diet" is of low diet quality and a "traditional diet" is of higher diet quality.

Another study, looking at the relationship of diet to mood in adults is titled "Dietary pattern and depressive symptoms in middle age." This work followed more than 3000 participants over a five-year time interval whose dietary habits fell into one of two categories:

> " 'whole food' (heavily loaded by vegetables, fruits and fish) and 'processed food' (heavily loaded by sweetened desserts, fried food, processed meat, refined grains and high-fat dairy products)."

At the end of the five years, depressive symptomatology was measured by a selected instrument called "CES-D". The conclusion was that:

> "In middle-aged participants, a processed food dietary pattern is a risk factor for CES–D depression 5 years later, whereas a whole food pattern is protective."

Within the limitations of the study, these results are statistically significant and rather dramatic.

Another large and recent prospective cohort study performed at the University College London showed a significant correlation between a healthy diet and the lack of depressive symptoms in women over a five-year time interval.

A "healthy diet" was based on the Harvard Alternative Healthy Eating Index, which emphasizes vegetables and fruits, low fat and limited oils, protein from sources such as fish, nuts, and seeds; it does, however, allow for inclusion of meat and dairy but less than the current USDA recommendations. Depressive symptoms were based on the Center for Epidemiologic Studies' Depression Scale.

The conclusion was that:

"there was a suggestion that a poor diet is a risk factor for future depression in women."

There was a positive dose-response nature as well, i.e., the healthier the diet the less the probability of developing sustained depressive symptoms over the five-year interval.

There are a number of other studies that make similar claims of improving mood in adults with better dietary patterns, such as a study performed at the University of Delaware, reported in 2010, which concludes:

"Diet quality was significantly associated with reported symptoms of depression."

And another at the University of Calgary in 2012 stating that their study :

"was consistent with prior epidemiologic surveys, revealing an association between higher levels of nutrient intakes and better mental health."

One particularly well-studied dietary pattern considered by some as a "healthy diet" is the *Mediterranean Diet*. This diet was inspired by the traditional dietary patterns of Greece, Spain and Southern Italy. These countries are the biggest olive producing countries, so it is no wonder that the diet features olive oil.

The principal aspects of this diet include proportionally high consumption of olive oil, legumes, unrefined cereals, fruits and vegetables, moderate to high consumption of fish, moderate consumption of dairy products, moderate wine consumption, and low consumption of meat and meat products.

This particular diet has been chosen for a number of psychiatric studies because the lifetime prevalence of mental disorders has been found to be lower in Mediterranean countries than in Northern European countries. Suicide rates, which may reflect the prevalence of severe depression, also tend to be lowest in Mediterranean countries.

One such study of the Mediterranean Diet, published in 2009 by a group at a Spanish university, examined over 10,000 participants using physicians' clinical diagnoses of mood disorder and the extent of adherence to the Mediterranean Diet over an average time interval of more than four years. They conclude that results:

> *"suggest a potential protective role of the Mediterranean Diet with regard to the prevention of depressive disorders."*

Another large prospective cohort epidemiologic investigation was reported recently by researchers at Loma Linda University. Their conclusion was that:

> *"foods typical of Mediterranean diets were associated with positive affect as well as lower negative affect while Western foods were associated with low positive affect in general and negative affect in women."*

All the studies shown so far in the context of exploring mood states define dietary patterns in various ways but allow various amounts of most all foods. What about more restrictive diets such as vegetarian or vegan? Few studies exist.

Bonnie Beezhold and colleagues at Arizona State University conducted such a study, but their motivation was the notion that vegetarian diets might harm brain function and mood states because they exclude fish, the major dietary source of *eicosapentaenoic acid* and *docosahexaenoic acid*, critical regulators of brain cell structure and function.

The investigators used a food frequency questionnaire and a psychometric test called the Depression Anxiety Stress Scale in a cross-sectional study.

The conclusion was that:

> *"The vegetarian diet profile does not appear to adversely affect mood despite low intake of long-chain omega-3 fatty acids."*

But the conclusion doesn't tell their whole story. Not only did the vegetarian diet not compromise mood states, results indicated a considerable advantage over an omnivore's diet for both females and males.

The same researchers more recently reported a similar study but in this one patients were randomly selected to receive three different diets over a two-week time interval: typical omnivore, omnivore with only fish as the flesh food, and vegetarian.

Their conclusion was that:

> *"Restricting meat, fish, and poultry improved some domains of short-term mood state in modern omnivores."*

And they are correct to point out the remarkable fact that:

> *"this is the first trial to examine the impact of restricting meat, fish, and poultry on mood state in omnivores."*

Their study has some additional interesting results – the effect on anxiety. The randomly selected individuals who ate the vegetarian diet happened to score the highest in anxiety level at the beginning of the study but scored the lowest compared to those on the other diets after two weeks.

The same was true with a measure of fatigue: the group with the vegetarian diet was worst at the beginning and best at the end of the study.

No dietary studies exist to date on what might be considered optimal diets of whole plant-based diets.

Teen dietary patterns – junk food, junk moods

Teen consumption of "junk foods" and other unhealthy dietary choices may be contributing significantly to the burgeoning mental health crisis in that age group.

Significant increases in the prevalence of adolescent emotional distress and behavioral problems have occurred over the past several generations.

Paralleling this mental health pathology among young people is a reduction in the quality of adolescents' diets over recent generations with decreasing consumption of raw fruits and high-nutrient vegetables and associated increases in consumption of fast food, snacks, and sweetened beverages with resulting obesity.

While data are still relatively scarce from randomized, controlled trials to demonstrate the efficacy of healthful eating on psychiatric disorders, there is considerable epidemiologic evidence. Most of that literature is based on studies of adults; however, emerging evidence suggests similar correlations with adolescent diets.

Cross-sectional studies indicate an association between dietary patterns and mental health in adolescence. Poorer emotional states and behavior were seen in adolescents with a typical Western dietary pattern high in red and processed meats, takeaway foods, confectionary and refined foods compared to those who consumed more fresh fruit and vegetables.

The first prospective cohort study on the effect of diet quality on mental health of adolescents was published in 2011, based on over 3000 adolescents 11 - 18 years old. Participants with poor diet quality at baseline had more emotional and behavioral problems; these worsened with time if a poor diet continued but improved if their diets improved. Those with good baseline diet quality had fewer psychiatric problems but if that diet deteriorated, so did their mental health. A healthy diet was defined as one that included fruit and vegetables as "core food groups" and included two or more servings of fruit per day and four or more servings of vegetables, as well as general avoidance of processed foods including chips, fried foods, chocolate, sweets, and ice cream.

In October 2013, results from a very large prospective cohort study of 20,000 women and their young children indicated that early poor nutritional exposures in utero were related to risk for behavioral and emotional problems in their children. These difficulties were more severe if the child's dietary pattern after birth was also poor.

The mechanisms behind these effects in children and adolescents are not well described.

Beyond the obvious neurological development in utero, we know that neurologic development continues after birth and extends throughout childhood and adolescence into young adulthood. It therefore appears logical that a highly nutrient-dense diet could result in an advantage in brain development with cognitive, emotional, and behavioral implications.

This could be an effect additional to the influence diet has on the mental health of adults through inflammation and the immune system, oxidative stress, and neurotrophic factors. A focus on psychiatric disorders in childhood and adolescence is particularly important given the fact that three quarters of lifetime psychiatric disorders will first emerge by late adolescence or early adulthood.

There appears to be a multitude of reasons why judicious choice of dietary patterns is important to establish early.

Therefore, in all practices of medicine regardless of specialization, it is important to include nutritional habits in assessments of children, adolescents, and adults. Dietary advice and education enhances physical and mental health.

We all wish long healthy lives but also happiness. Good foods are integral to good moods.

Chapter Seven

The New Ancestral Diet

"Don't dig your grave with your own knife and fork."

English Proverb

All nutrients, macronutrients, micronutrients, and phytonutrients come from plants reacting with the sun. If we eat animals or animal products, they may or may not have the nutrients we need but they have a lot of compounds we don't want.

We have indicated from an analysis of the past 85 million years of primate history how we have been primarily whole-food plant-based during the vast percentage of that time. Only very recently in our history as a species have we resorted to eating energy - dense animals, first by scavenging organs and marrow and then, after control of fire, occasionally cooking and consuming flesh.

We have seen that genetic metabolic changes occurred in our direct ancestors tens of millions of years ago including losing the ability to self-manufacture the essential micronutrients:

- thiamine
- riboflavin
- niacin
- vitamin A
- vitamin C

Also, over thousands of millennia we lost the ability to produce the following substances:

- alpha gal
- Neu5Gc

Unfortunately, the animals which are consumed today still do produce these substances, are involved in chronic inflammation and autoimmune disorders, including cancers.

We know that meat contains bacteria that produce endotoxins that are taken up by our bodies, contributing to chronic inflammation - the leading cause of morbidity and mortality in Western societies.

We know that meat contains mostly "bad fats" (for example trans-fat and saturated fat) that is added to our own fat virtually unchanged - "lips to hips".

We know that meat products contain cholesterol, a compound that is made in sufficient quantities in our own bodies but dietary intake can directly lead to vascular disease, including heart failure and strokes.

There is yet another analogous substance that we make in our own bodies, as do all animals, but do not want contributions from animals that we consume: arachidonic acid. Arachidonic acid is a key substrate for the synthesis of proinflammatory compounds that can adversely affect mental health via a cascade of neuroinflammation.

Caloric macronutrient distribution

We have seen that throughout the great majority of our evolution as primates, we have adopted a whole-food plant-based diet.

Let's explore the ideal distribution of macronutrients with recommendations from science today.

The National Academy of Sciences Institute of Medicine's Food and Nutrition Board gives the following information for macronutrient composition:

Macronutrient	AMDR, % calories
Carbohydrate	45 - 65
Fat	20 - 35
Protein	10 - 35

The *Acceptable Macronutrient Distribution Range* (AMDR) given for carbohydrates is relatively low as it is assumed that up to 25% of calories are from simple, refined, processed sugars. As this is not the case when eating whole fruits and vegetables, we shall set a suggested 75%.

The AMDR given for fat is somewhat high to adjust for the carbohydrate percentage being rather low. This includes the essential omega-3 and omega-6 polyunsaturated fatty acids. Saturated fats, trans fats and cholesterol, always present in significant quantities in animal products, is not recommended at any level. The presence of some fats increases the absorption of fat-soluble vitamins and precursors such as vitamin A and pro-vitamin A carotenoids. We will favor a daily fat intake of 10%, assuming there is no substantial need for additional fat storage.

For protein, we will suggest a lower-range AMDR of 15%. The nine essential amino acids must be present in the diet.

With these allotments for the daily intake of macronutrients, the distribution is given in the following pie chart, in relative percent calories.

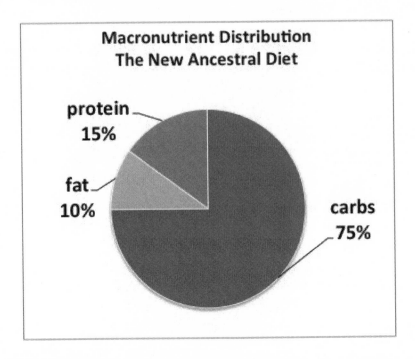

This distribution is consistent with that suggested, for example, by Neal Barnard of the Physicians Committee for Responsible Medicine for a whole-food plant-based diet that primates have subsisted on throughout their evolution, including the great majority of the Paleolithic Period.

While some may argue that 15% protein is too low, consider the fact that human breast milk, a whole-food complete diet composition designed by nature as most nourishing, contains only 8% of its total calories as protein.

It is perhaps useful to note that a leafy green food such as kale has a macronutrient composition of 73% carbohydrates, 12% fat, and 15% protein, closely approximating our suggested ideal.

The Okinawa traditional diet

People of the Okinawa archipelago in Japan have the nutritionally dense traditional diet of that region – they also have one of the highest longevity rates in the world.

Their macronutrient mix is shown in the following pie chart:

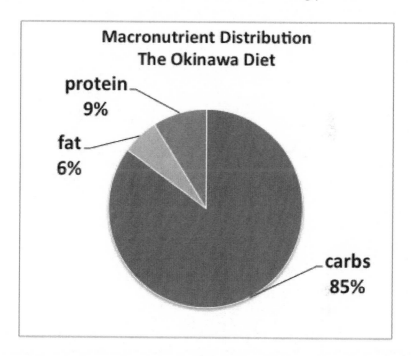

In addition to their long life expectancy, islanders are noted for their low mortality from cardiovascular disease (eight times less than Americans) and certain types of cancers, such as prostate, breast, and colon cancers.

Other factors in addition to diet undoubtedly contribute to the longevity of Okinawan centenarians. Most grew a garden, a source of daily physical activity as well as fresh organic vegetables. Tending a garden also lowers stress and increases vitamin D intake.

Standard American Diet (SAD)

The National Health and Nutrition Examination Survey is the primary national data system which provides information to monitor the nutritional status of the U.S. population. The macronutrient distribution is shown below:

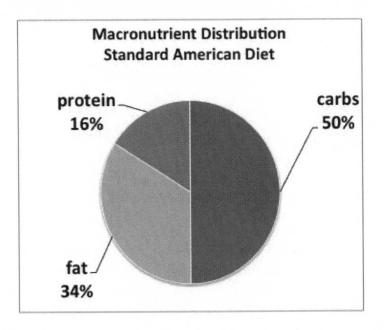

The suggested macronutrient distribution of the New Ancestral Diet is closer to the Okinawa Diet than to the Standard American Diet, the SAD being lower in total carbohydrates but high in refined sugar and containing more than three times the fat content. This is shown in the following RAM graphic:

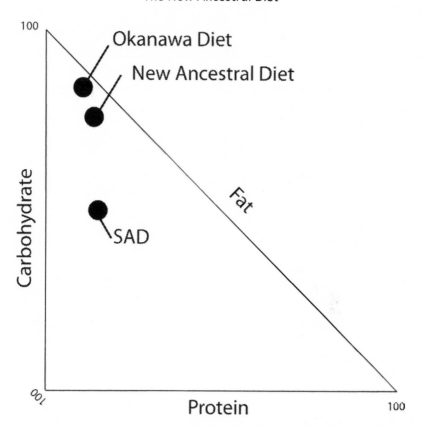

Energy density versus nutrient density

As has been detailed, the main activity of our ancestral primates has been eating – acquiring calories for energy. Energy-dense foods, therefore, have been favored to assure adequate caloric intake.

This is no longer an issue in Western society from a food availability standpoint. Nevertheless, energy-density is still favored in the *Standard American Diet* (SAD) over *nutrient density*.

Consider the following graph title "Food Quality" on which energy density and nutrient density are indicated for a number of different foods. "Percent max" on the ordinate is based on pure fat as 100% energy dense; percent max for nutrient density is based on the measure used by Nutrition Data.

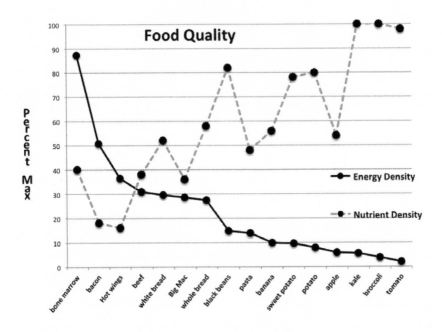

Generally there is an inverse relationship between energy density and nutrient density.

Those foods favored by the SAD include those of highest energy density such as bacon, hot wings, beef, and the Big Mac. Those of the highest nutrient density include tomatoes, broccoli, and kale.

A choice of foods based on cut-off points for these two parameters might be: energy density less than 20% and nutrient density greater than 40%. That effectively eliminates animal products and refined grains.

The graph below illustrates the ratio of nutrient content (as defined above) to energy density for select fruits and vegetables.

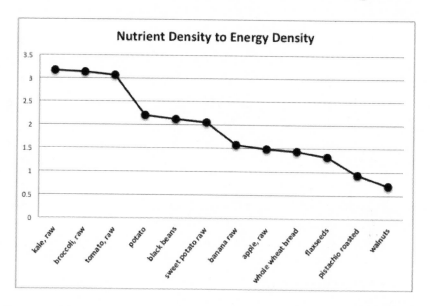

There can be seen on the plot a couple of plateaus: the first, at the highest ratio, contains typical green vegetables; the second, legumes and underground storage organs; then fruits; and finally grains, seeds, and nuts. Basically, this is the order of priority we recommend when constructing a daily menu.

Yes, but where do vegans get their protein?

No question is asked more frequently of vegans than this one. The answer is "from a whole-food plant-based varied diet." Consider the largest study of nutrient composition ever conducted on about 30,000 non-vegetarians, 20,000 vegetarians and about 5,000 vegans. Even considering a rather large average daily intake of 42 gm per day, omnivores got way more protein than this – and so did the vegetarians and vegans, roughly 70% more than they required each day.

There is virtually no one with a protein deficiency in the Western world. But there is a large deficiency in other food components. Fiber, for example.

Fiber

Fiber, although not considered a macronutrient, has an RDA of 25 – 38 gm/day, again according to the National Academy of Sciences Institute of Medicine's Food and Nutrition Board and is only available from plants. And we know that the most healthful diet is one that is high in fiber and low in rapidly digested carbohydrates. This regimen is referred to as a *low-glycemic* diet because it helps keep our blood glucose at optimum levels. Wild fruits and vegetables are the original low-glycemic foods.

It is estimated that 97% of Americans do not consume the recommended minimum amount of fiber.

Shown below are a few example foods and their fiber density, expressed as grams of fiber per total grams of dry weight of food substance.

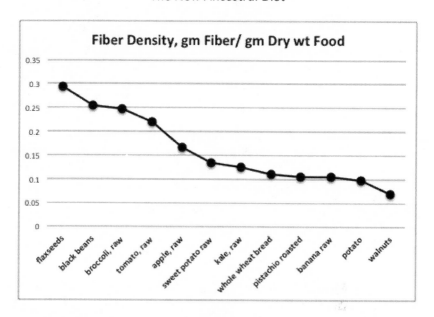

Generalizing, fruits and vegetables are significant sources of fiber, but beans and cruciferous vegetables are best, and starch and grains much less so.

Omega-3 fatty acids

Omega-3 fatty acids are *polyunsaturated fatty acids* (PUFAs) hydrocarbon chains with one end labeled *alpha* and the other end *omega*. The "poly" in polyunsaturated means "many" and unsaturated means there are double carbon bonds so taken together these fatty acids have many carbon double bonds. The "3" in omega-3 refers to the first double bond from the omega end occuring at the third carbon.

That's all unnecessary for you to know except this molecule is so important that the name should be a little more real to you now.

There are three types of omega-3 fatty acids:

- *α-linolenic acid* (ALA)
- eicosapentaenoic acid (EPA)
- docosahexaenoic acid (DHA)

Of these three, only ALA is *essential* because it can lead to synthesis of EPA and then subsequently to DHA.   ALA is manufactured by all plants, likely having a regulatory function; it is abundant in seeds, particularly flaxseeds. An *adequate intake* (AI) for ALA is 1.6 grams/day for men and 1.1 grams/day for women. This can be easily obtained with a whole-food plant-based varied diet. About one teaspoon of flaxseeds contains the daily AI (be certain to crush or grind).

Fish oils have been popularized as an omega-3 supplemental option. However, the omega-3s found in fish oils (EPA and DHA) are actually highly unstable molecules that tend to decompose and unleash dangerous free radicals, making these supplements an unfavorable option. In addition, current research demonstrates that taking fish oil supplements does not actually produce significant protection of cardiovascular health. And such supplements, being processed and non-whole food extracts from fish livers, introduces the unknowns of what additional oils and potential toxins might be present.

Research has shown that omega-3s are found in the more stable form, ALA, in vegetables, fruits, and beans. In fact, according to a European Prospective Investigation into Cancer and Nutrition, women on vegan diets actually have more EPA and DHA in their blood compared with fish-eaters, meat-eaters, and lacto-ovo vegetarians.

Omega-6 to omega-3 ratio

Omega-6s are pro-inflammatory, while Omega-3s have an anti-inflammatory effect.

We evolved genetic patterns established on a diet with a ratio of omega-6 to omega-3 essential fatty acids (EFA) of approximately 1 whereas in Western diets the ratio is about 16. This high ratio promotes the pathogenesis of vascular disease, cancer, and inflammatory and autoimmune diseases, whereas lower ratios exert suppressive effects. For example, in the secondary prevention of cardiovascular disease, a ratio of 4/1 was associated with a 70% decrease in total mortality.

A distorted ratio of these polyunsaturated fatty acids may be one of the most damaging aspects of the Western diet.

The plot below illustrates the ratio of omega-3 to omega-6 for some select foods.

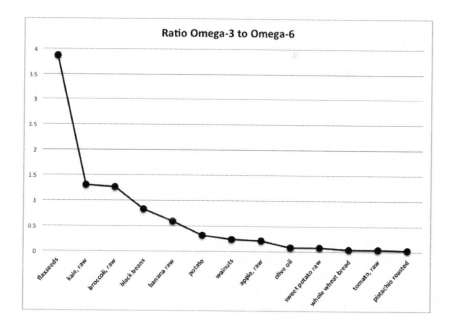

Typical green vegetables contain the ratio experienced by our primate ancestors. Legumes are acceptable sources for these essential fats as well. Flaxseeds have an extraordinarily favorable content of these nutrients and can be used in small quantities to assure adequate intake (a teaspoon crushed in a smoothie or on salad, as examples).

Wild edibles

"Weeds are flowers too, once you get to know them".
Eeyore from Winnie the Pooh

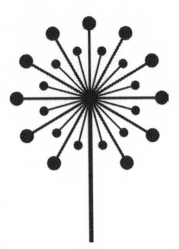

There are plants that grow wild and have not been modified by humans for domestication, yet are nontoxic and provide a full complement of macro- and micro-nutrients. Such plants have an excellent likelihood of containing a strong spectrum of phytonutrients. They tend to be higher on the bitterness spectrum or present a textural element that some consider unpleasant.

dandelions – bet you can't eat just one

Dandelions are found worldwide. They are thought to have evolved about thirty million years ago. They are considered a noxious weed and a nuisance in residential and recreational lawns in North America; however, they are entirely edible – flower, stem, leaves, and roots. Although there are records of human consumption of dandelions, the degree of bitterness of each part of the plant renders them discouraging to eat. Perhaps this is reflected in the various other names it is known by, for example, *piss-a-bed* , *worm rose*, and *cankerwort*.

Dandelion leaves contain abundant vitamins and minerals, especially vitamins A, C, and K, and are good sources of calcium, potassium, iron, and manganese. They have significant anti-inflammatory, anti-oxidative, anti-carcinogenic, analgesic, anti-hyperglycemic, anti-coagulatory, and prebiotic effects. Wild dandelion leaves, once a springtime treat for Native Americans, compared to spinach have eight times more antioxidants, a higher content of dietary fiber and proteins, a greater variety of amino acids, vitamins, and minerals, and have higher proportions of unsaturated fatty acids (oleic, palmitoleic, linoleic, and linolenic).

Emerging scientific evidence suggests that dandelions might have potential to prevent or ameliorate the outcome of several degenerative diseases such as atherosclerosis, coronary artery and vascular disease, obesity, diabetes mellitus, and cancer.

So the irony is that this highly nutritious omnipresent plant is deselected from growing near our homes in preference to non-edible other plant varieties (lawn grasses) that are groomed weekly. This superior plant is poisoned or ripped out of our lawns and placed into the trash.

purslane

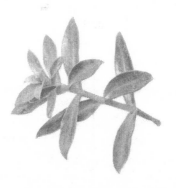

Considered a weed in the United States, purslane is a nutritious leafy vegetable. The stems, leaves, and flower buds are all edible. Purslane contains more omega-3 fatty acids than any other leafy vegetable, including 0.01 mg/g of EPA. It also contains a variety of vitamins and minerals with six times more vitamin E than spinach and seven times more beta-carotene than carrots.

Archaeobotanical finds of purslane are common at many prehistoric sites, so our ancestors likely ate this plant in the wild. It's unclear if there has been domestication of varieties of this plant, but it is dense with phytonutrients. Two types of red and yellow pigments are potent antioxidants and have been found in laboratory studies to have antimutagenic properties.

stinging nettle

It's the texture that discourages animals – including humans - from eating this nutritious plant with tiny needles that inject the inflammatory molecule histamine; interestingly, they also inject small quantities of the human neurotransmitters acetylcholine and serotonin.

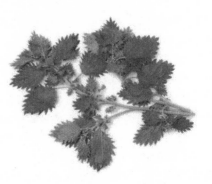

Nettles are quite edible, however, and rich in vitamins and minerals. Soaking nettles in water or cooking removes the stinging chemicals from the plant. They contain 25% (dry weight) protein, some of the highest protein content for a leafy green vegetable.

Food processing

Although the nature of fruits and vegetables has likely changed considerably over the years with domestication, selection of mutations favorable to convenience, taste/flavor, and hybridization, there remains the same challenge of to ancestors of dealing with the fibrous content, that is, all the chewing.

Without resorting to "pre-processing" by the food industry, there are several techniques that assist with this problem.

crushing

One method of processing fiber developed in the Stone Age is crushing plants between two stones. We use the mortar and pestle shown here.

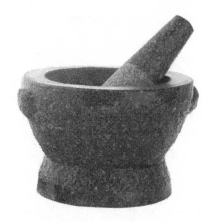

Our initial use was specifically for making pesto using basil, garlic, walnuts, nutritional yeast, and sea salt. However, now its use has expanded to making a variety of pestos, including the ultimate one described in the Appendix.

We have a 3+ cup capacity 8-inch diameter stone from a single block of granite. It is practically indestructible – will not chip or crack even under vigorous pounding (Mohs scale 7+). It's also rather beautiful. Cost was $34 online on Amazon.com.

blending

Even more popular in our household is mechanical blending. We use a Vitamix Turboblend VS shown here; with almost two horsepower, it will blend any food to a smooth texture. Most mornings, we prepare a "green smoothie," primarily containing three to six cups of green leafy vegetables

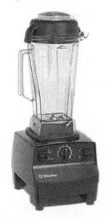

that would require a great deal of chewing otherwise. To this is added various other vegetables from our garden or from the farmers' market. The bitterness factor is modulated by the addition of fruit. Typically we use fresh frozen organic fruit as this allows a nice varied inventory and adds a refreshing chill to the drink.

We always add a tablespoon of flaxseeds and another of dried shredded hibiscus flowers. Rather than drink the water extract of herbal teas in general, we occasionally add the whole plant to our smoothies - rooibos, green teas, etc. All teas can be bought in bulk much less expensively than in marketed tea bag form.

Other items can easily be added for a *super smoothie* such as fenugreek seeds, cacao, cinnamon, maca roots, dried hot peppers, cordyceps – obviously any food of your choice.

We drink these smoothies for their nutritional content and don't worry too much about the taste. This is the true Ancestral Diet way – eating for survival.

We typically make plenty of smoothie so that after consuming a nice big glass for breakfast, we fill a blender bottle (shown here) and take it on the road or to work, placing it in a cooler; we use a bag with ice wraps intended for keeping a baby bottle cool. Then through the morning or afternoon, we distribute the nutrients with a swallow 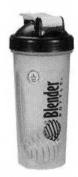 periodically. This keeps the hunger at bay all day while *bio-hacking* nutrition distribution and bioavailability.

cooking

This is a must for root vegetables. Potatoes and sweet potatoes are not adequately digested without cooking. Other plants become easier to chew and can obtain an acceptable blend of flavors through cooking.

There are many ways to cook, basically applying heat to effect chemical changes. Roasting applies primarily dry radiated heat. Our favorite is hearth cooking – placing vegetables on the hearth near a wood burning fire. This can be done also on the grill, although the danger of charring increases. Roasting can enhance flavor through caramelization and Maillard browning on the surface of the food.

A very promising cooking method for vegetables is sous-vide in which the vegetable is placed into an airtight plastic bag in a temperature-controlled water bath for a precise amount of time. The bath is typically of low cooking temperature, such as 130 degrees Fahrenheit, and requires an hour or two of cooking time. Carrots, one of the few vegetables that increase their nutrition with cooking, when cooked sous-vide retain the natural sweetness, bright color, and firm bite that often are in traditional cooking. Blanching, for example, dilutes the carrots' natural sugars, making them bland, while boiling tends to make them mushy. Cooking sous-vide prevents overcooking and helps retain color, texture, and flavor.

Bottom lines

Eat fresh whole plants in as large a variety as you can. Give preference to vegetables low in starch and fat. Process by chewing, crushing, blending, or cooking. Go easy on grains, nuts and seeds. Allow no processed foods whatsoever, including no oils.

If you have the space, grow a garden. Particularly, a variety of leafy vegetables is easy to grow and they regenerate quickly after frequent harvesting. Heritage seeds are available that may maximize nutrition and flavor.

Eat like a primate!

Appendix

EPIC STONE AGE MEAL

Q: *"How does it taste?"*

A: *"It tastes nutritious."*

This is a question and answer often heard in our household.

Most meals that we prepare are intended to optimize nutrition, consistent with the theme of this book, returning to the idea of eating to survive. We don't spend much time attempting to make food "taste good" in the usual sense of being sweet (less bitter) or savory. Instead, we have learned to associate food preparations with health, and even if they taste bitter, we enjoy the association with health and "like" the taste.

The result may or may not be "delicious" but is definitely "nutritious".

Blending

For example, most mornings we prepare a green smoothie – it's always a little different as the ingredients vary – different fruits and vegetables and relative quantities of each, although a lot of green leafys. Also, what is used very much depends on what happens to be in the garden or the refrigerator.

We include fruit, usually fresh frozen organic berries which balance the bitterness from the green leaves. We add lemon or lime as an antioxidant.

Again, there is no recipe - whatever is "gathered" from the garden and refrigerator. We like this ancestral association, even if a remote one.

We do like the smoothie smooth and cool, so ice is added and blending is at high speeds in the Vitamix for at least 30 seconds.

There will ultimately be suspended solids, so the product is consumed immediately after blending. Try to allow pretty good contact and swirl a mouthful somewhat like a fine wine in order to allow pre-digestive processes to occur before swallowing.

Enough smoothie is made for consumption later that day as well, to gradually introduce nutrition throughout the day. In the interest of keeping the drink smooth and cool, the remaining drink is poured into a blender bottle and stored in the baby bottle cooler mentioned in Chapter Seven. The blender bottle is given a brisk shake prior to taking a drink.

The Stone Age way

We do appreciate texture somewhat so there are certain vegetables that we rarely blend but rather consume in a different manner. These include USOs such as sweet potatoes, onions, and garlic; also beans and grains.

We try always to include *lots* of green leafy vegetables with every meal. But there is the age-old (literally – for millions of years) dilemma of all that chewing of leaves. Blending is one way, but another supplements the texture issue nicely when eating USOs, grains, and beans: stone crushing.

The epic meal

We would like to give you one detailed specific "recipe", although would not suggest one follow this precisely because it doesn't make that much of a difference. We really never exactly reproduce any meal. But the overall method and the ingredients are recommended.

First, here is our little home garden (or half of it) - seen are primarily green leafy vegetables that can be continuously harvested all spring, summer, and early fall. The beet greens in the foreground are harvested even before the beets themselves.

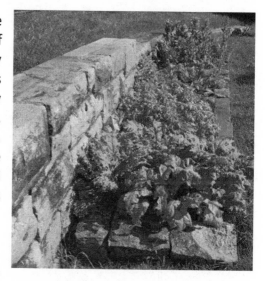

Much of what is grown we start from seeds. We use heritage seeds from Baker Creek Heirloom Seed Company. The first ingredient from the garden was kale. Each ingredient was weighed so as to provide a precise nutritional summary. Here is the scale weighing a portion of the kale, 17 grams worth.

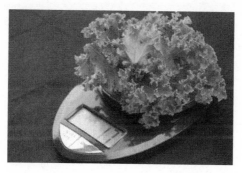

The total amount of kale used, 130 grams, is shown here in the mortar - on the left before crushing and on the right, after exactly 5 minutes of crushing. You can see the tough leaves are considerably reduced in volume to a paste.

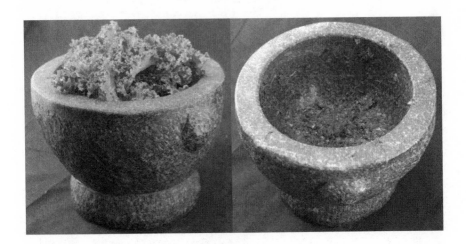

Next are shown the following leafy green ingredients from the garden, left to right, top to bottom: arugula, 25 gm; greens from the heritage beet plant "Early Wonder," pre-1811, 41 gm; basil, 26 gm; and dandelion, 12 gm.

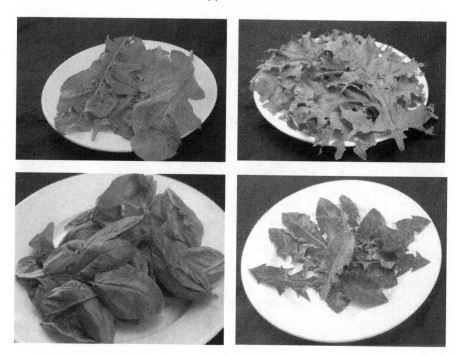

Also added to the mortar were garlic cloves, 16 gm; flaxseeds, 4 g; freshly crushed black pepper, 0.5 gm; and a slice of lemon with peel, 23 gm.

These ingredients were crushed for about 7 minutes. Next, freshly sprouted buckwheat, 64 gm, was added. The mixture at this stage is shown here.

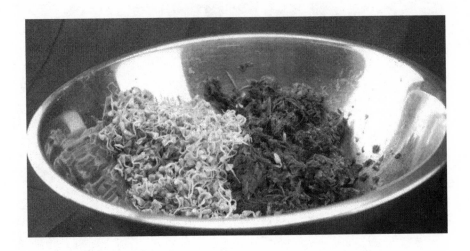

Organically grown black beans were soaked in water overnight to begin the sprouting process, then slowly cooked the previous day. Here is shown about one and a half cups, 245 gm.

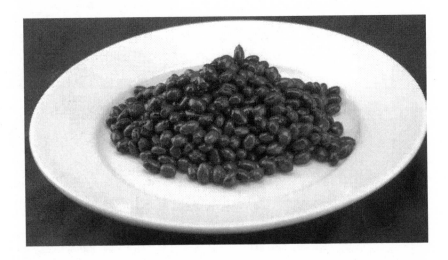

This recipe provides two servings, one shown here.

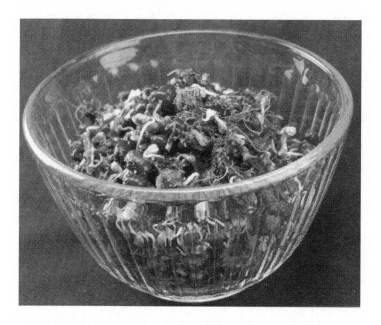

Analysis

The total weight of this combination of food is 592.5 gm; it results in 648.2 calories. The breakdown in calories is:

- carbohydrates: 71%
- protein: 19%
- fat: 10%

This is approximately the ideal caloric distribution given in Chapter Seven; it is a little higher in protein because of the black beans. There is 31.8 gm of fiber, 3.0 gm omega-3, and 1.7 gm omega-6.

Most importantly, it is very high in phytonutrients.

How does it taste?

We knew you'd ask! We fully expected it to taste "nutritious."
We asked family member Quinton, who is more critical than we
concerning food taste, to try the first bite. His summary:

"It tastes delicious!"

References

Chapter One
Plants as Animals

Common origins

"Miller-Urey" graduate student experiments: Miller, S. (1953). A Production of Amino Acids Under Possible Primitive Earth Conditions. *Science, 117*(3046), 528-529.

...spontaneous generation à la   Aristotle: Balme, D. (1962). Development of Biology in Aristotle and Theophrastus: Theory of Spontaneous Generation. *Phronesis: A Journal for Ancient Philosophy, 7*(1-2), 91-104.

Supercell

...the common ancestor for all of life past and present: Futuyma, D. (2005). *Evolution.* Sunderland, Massachusetts: Sinauer Associates.

Bacteria can survive almost everywhere on the planet, from the coldest to the hottest places on earth, to the bottom of the oceans, in radioactive waste: Fredrickson, J., Zachara, J., Balkwill, D., Kennedy, D., Li, S., Kostandarithes, H., . . . Brockman, F. (2004). Geomicrobiology of High-Level Nuclear Waste-Contaminated Vadose Sediments at the Hanford Site, Washington State. *Applied and Environmental Biology, 70*(7), 4230-4241.

No other organism is as adaptable: Amyes, S. (2013). Very Short Introductions. In *Bacteria: A Very Short Introduction* (p. Xiii). Oxford University Press.

It's complicated

The eukaryote is defined and differentiated from the prokaryote mainly as an organism consisting of a cell in which the genetic material is DNA in the form of chromosomes contained within a distinct nucleus.

We have derived a mathematical proof of this principle for the simple, widely used predator-prey ecological model elsewhere: Aiken, R.C., and Lapidus, L. (1973). The stability of interacting populations. *International Journal of Systems Science. 4 (4), 691-695.* This was my first publication as a graduate student at Princeton University; it was perhaps the first non-linear differential equation set to be proven stable "in the round", i.e. regardless of the initial conditions.

Franken cells

...recent genome sequencing: Gray, M.W. (1998). Rickettsia, typhus and the mitochondrial connection. *Nature. 396, 109-110.*

After it was "eaten" or otherwise introduced into the eukaryotic cell. This process is termed *endiocytosis.*

Another perhaps even *more* profound example of cellular survival of mutually beneficial organisms happened about a billion years ago, give or take a few hundred million years: Mcfadden, G., & Dooren, G. (2004). Evolution: Red Algal Genome Affirms a Common Origin of All Plastids. *Current Biology, 14*(13).

...the *chloroplast*, a cell within the eukaryotic cell which provides photosynthetic production of energy from sunlight: Recent electron micrographs have shown a glimpse at how scientists think early organisms acquired free-living chloroplasts, which helped raise oxygen levels in Earth's atmosphere and paved the way for the rise of animals. See Maruyama, S., & Kim, E. (2012). A Modern Descendant of Early Green Algal Phagotrophs. *Current Biology, 23*(12), 1081-1084.

...the last common ancestor (LCA) was probably much before, at about 1.6 billion years ago: Meyerowitz, E. (2002). Plants Compared to Animals: The Broadest Comparative Study of Development. *Science, 295*(5559), 1482-1485.

One might argue that plants need aerobic species to provide carbon dioxide, but this was untrue before the emergence of significant numbers of aerobic organisms and its concentration is determined by geothermal processes, not respiration.

Common sense

This life process ultimately requires energy and mass combining in an electrochemical reaction: The primary source of energy is our star, the sun, the only other energy source being the fissionable materials generated by the death of other stars prior to the formation of Earth as a planet. These fissionable materials trapped in Earth's crust is what gives rise to geothermal energy, which drives the volcanism on Earth and also makes it possible for humans to fuel nuclear reactors.

Beyond all else as living entities, we must *eat:* Maslow, A. (1943). A theory of human motivation. *Psychological Review, 50*(4), 370-396.

Plants land first

Land plants evolved on earth by about 700 million years ago through a team effort by lichens and green algae in receding shallow pools of water: Maruyama, S., & Kim, E. (2012). A Modern Descendant of Early Green Algal Phagotrophs. *Current Biology, 23*(12), 1081-1084.

This wall is made of cellulose: Although some animals, particularly ruminants and termites, can digest cellulose with the help of symbiotic micro-organisms that live in their guts and even humans can digest cellulose to a minor extent, it is often referred to as "dietary fiber".

More than half of all terrestrial biomass is composed of cellulose: Robert, D., & Rowland, J. (1989). Biologie Vegetale: Characteristiques et Strategie Evolutive des Plantes. Organisation Cellulaire.

Fortunately for us all, plants have a rate of energy capture by photosynthesis that is enormous: *Net primary production* is the rate at which all the plants in an ecosystem produce net useful chemical energy; it is equal to the difference between the rate at which the plants in an ecosystem produce useful chemical energy and the rate at which they use some of that energy during respiration. Some net primary production goes toward growth and reproduction of plants producing it, while the rest is a potential food source for predatory herbivores.

...which is about six times greater than the current power consumption of human civilization: Nealson, K., & Conrad, P. (1999). Life: Past, present and future. *Philosophical Transactions of the Royal Society B: Biological Sciences, 354*(1392), 1923-1939.

...mitochondria convert into an energy currency called *ATP* later at night, or at other times when the sun is not available: This is a simple but brilliant solution to the storage issue plaguing most solar energy schemes. We were part of an experiment to overcome the limitations of solar energy production onboard the space shuttle. Energy was readily available during the 45-minute daytime, but once the sun was behind the earth, energy had to be obtained from solar energy stored onboard using heavy lead batteries. To remedy this, we constructed the largest armature motor in the world – or around the world – consisting of a 12-mile long electrodynamic tether that was thrown out of the cargo bay, as by a huge fishing reel. The tether was a conducting medium and as it traversed the earth's magnetic field, this induced an electric current for onboard use. Unfortunately, the drag on the cable even in the rarified atmosphere was enough to remove any net gains in energy production. The Tethered Satellite System-1 (TSS-1) was proposed by NASA and the Italian Space Agency (ASI) in the early 1970s by Mario Grossi, of the Smithsonian Astrophysical Observatory, and Giuseppe Colombo, of Padua University. A joint NASA-Italian Space Agency project, it was flown during STS-46 aboard the Space Shuttle Atlantis from July 31 to August 8, 1992. We were involved in the mathematical modeling and computer simulation analysis of that experiment.

Animals as plants

There is considerable evidence that these basic and critical immune defenses have ancient origins: Medzhitov, R., & Janeway,, C. (2000). Innate Immunity. *N. Engl. J. Med, 343*, 338-344.

...a consequence of *convergent* evolution and reflect inherent constraints on how an innate immune system can be constructed: Ausubel, F. (2005). Are innate immune signaling pathways in plants and animals conserved? *Nature Immunology, 6*(10), 973-979.

...such plant compounds serve as a stimulating factor for human active immune response: Nishi, K., Kondo, A., Okamoto, T., Nakano, H., Daifuku, M., Nishimoto, S., . . . Sugahara, T. (2011). Immunostimulatory in Vitro and in Vivo Effects of a Water-Soluble Extract from Kale. *Bioscience, Biotechnology and Biochemistry,* *75*(1), 40-46.

Chapter Two
Primal Primate Provisions

Acquiring a taste

... they are the targets of approximately 40% of all modern medicinal drugs: Filmore, D. (2004). It's a GPCR World. *Modern Drug Discovery (American Chemical Society)*, 24-28.

Not being bitter

Plant secondary compounds that have significant toxicity are typically bitter: Maga, J., & Rousseff, R. (1990). Compound Structure Versus Bitter Taste. *In Bitterness in Foods and Beverages: Developments in Food Science* (Vol. 25). Amsterdam: Elsevier.

Detection thresholds for bitter taste are extremely low in primates, whereas those for sugars are also low but very much higher than that of bitterness. Hladik, C., & Simmen, B. (1996). Taste perception and feeding behavior in nonhuman primates and human populations. *Evolutionary Anthropology: Issues, News, and Reviews Evol. Anthropol., 5,* 58-71.

This taste receptor gene set also is basic to whether a given species is an omnivore, herbivore, or carnivore. Caspermeyer, J. (2013). Avoiding Poisons: A Matter of Bitter Taste? *Molecular Biology and Evolution (Oxford University Press)*, 498-499.

Note that although we refer to "omnivores", there is no well-accepted definition of such animal species and one might more accurately think of herbivores or carnivores that have an extended ability to utilize sources of food that are of animal or plant origin, respectively.

The Tas2r genes in humans are thought to comprise about 25 different taste receptors, recognizing a wide variety of bitter-tasting compounds. Meyerhof, W., Batram, C., Kuhn, C., Brockhoff, A., Chudoba, E., Bufe, B., . . . Behrens, M. (2009). The Molecular Receptive Ranges of Human TAS2R Bitter Taste Receptors. *Chemical Senses, 35*(2), 157-170.

It has been speculated recently that inclusion of more animal products into human diets may be limiting the full expression of this family of genes responsible for sensitivity to bitterness. Wang, X. (2004). Relaxation of selective constraint and loss of function in the evolution of human bitter taste receptor genes. *Human Molecular Genetics, 13*(21), 2671-2678.

...over half of such human olfactory genes are nonfunctional. Gilad, Y., Man, O., Paabo, S., & Lancet, D. (2003). Human specific loss of olfactory receptor genes. *Proceedings of the National Academy of Sciences, 100*, 3324-3327.

While olfactory receptors representing "sniffing" or breathing in external environmental sensations have been deselected, those olfactory receptors posterior, sensitive to breathing out and flavor appreciation have become much more active recently.

...higher in protein and lower in fiber and toxins than mature leaves: Jones, S., Martin, R., & Pilbeam, D. (1994). *The Cambridge Encyclopedia of Human Evolution.* Cambridge: Cambridge University Press.

...unripe fruit typically contains more toxic compounds and has a higher degree of bitterness compared to fully ripened fruit: Glendinning, J. (1994). Is the bitter rejection response always adaptive? *Physiology & Behavior, 56,* 1217-1227.

...rise of plants bearing flowers and fleshy fruits: Simmen, B., & Hladik, C. (1993). Taste perception and adaptation to the nutritional environment in non human primates and human populations (Perception gustative et adaptation à l'environnement nutritionnel des Primates non-humains et des populations humaines). *Bulletins Et Mémoires De La Société D'anthropologie De Paris Bmsap,* 343-354.

...encouraging the utilization of a wide range of food items having a low sugar content yet perceived as edible: Hladik, C., Pasquet, P., & Simmen, B. (2002). New perspectives on taste and primate evolution: The dichotomy in gustatory coding for perception of beneficent versus noxious substances as supported by correlations among human thresholds. *Am. J. Phys. Anthropol. American Journal of Physical Anthropology,* 117, 342-348.

Bitter sweet

The pleasant taste response of saltiness very unlikely is based on genetic adaptation: Hladik, C., Pasquet, P., & Simmen, B. (2002). New perspectives on taste and primate evolution: The dichotomy in gustatory coding for perception of beneficent versus noxious substances as supported by correlations among human thresholds. *Am. J. Phys. Anthropol. American Journal of Physical Anthropology,* 117, 342-348.

85 MYA to 50 MYA

Rewinding to about 85 MYA, a type of mammal first classified as a *primate* diverged from the rest: Lee, M. (1999). Molecular Clock Calibrations and Metazoan Divergence Dates. *Journal of Molecular Evolution J Mol Evol, 49*(3), 385-391.

...weighing in at 2 lbs. or less, and eating a largely insectivorous diet: Andrews, Peter; Martin, Lawrence (1992) "Hominoid dietary evolution." In: Whiten A. and Widdowson E.M. (editors/organizers), *Foraging Strategies and Natural Diet of Monkeys, Apes, and Humans: Proceedings of a Royal Society Discussion Meeting held on 30 and 31 May, 1991.* Oxford, England: Clarendon Press. p. 41.

An approximate cutoff point of 500 grams (about one pound) has been suggested: Called *Kay's Threshold*, after the primatologist Richard Kay, who first proposed this.

Wild fruit, likely more similar to that eaten by our frugivoric cousins, differs considerably from cultivated fruit in that it contains much more fiber, pectin, protein, and micronutrients: Milton, K. (1999). Nutritional characteristics of wild primate foods: Do the diets of our closest living relatives have lessons for us? *Nutrition, 15,* 488-498.

It was faster on the ground than on the top of trees and began to spend longer times on lower branches feeding on fruits and leaves: Dawkins, R. (2004). *The Ancestor's Tale: A Pilgrimage to the Dawn of Evolution.* Boston: Houghton Mifflin.

Berry berry

Our increased ancestral reliance on fruits and vegetables led to the loss of the ability to produce the essential nutrient thiamine, also known as vitamin B_1: This began with the primates known as the "dry-nosed" primates, members of the clade Haplorhini, to which Old World monkeys, apes, and humans belong.

Nobel laureate Linus Pauling championed the theory: Perhaps this occurred even several hundred millions years ago, according to Linus Pauling, Evolution and the need for ascorbic acid. Proc Natl Acad Sci U S A. 1970 Dec;67(4):1643-8.

...must have lost the mechanism that allowed it to synthesize thiamine: Pauling, L. (1970). Evolution and the Need for Ascorbic Acid. *Proceedings of the National Academy of Sciences, 67*(4), 1643-1648.

...beriberi that affects primarily the peripheral nervous system causing suffering through heart disease and paralysis possibly leading to death: Mahan, L. (2000*). Krause's food, nutrition, & diet therapy* (10th ed.). Philadelphia: W.B. Saunders.

...nutrients that must be obtained through diet such as riboflavin, nicotinic acid, and vitamin A, supporting a very early reliance on plants as food sources: Pauling, L. (1970). Evolution and the Need for Ascorbic Acid. *Proceedings of the National Academy of Sciences, 67*(4), 1643-1648.

Amounts of vitamin C required to avoid disease from insufficient dietary intake of this substance: Scurvy is a disease resulting from lack of vitamin C, since without this vitamin, the synthesized collagen is too unstable to perform its function. A person with the ailment looks pale, feels depressed, and is lethargic. In advanced scurvy there are open wounds, loss of teeth and, eventually, death.

This is a water-soluble substance that cannot be stored for very long in the body: MedlinePlus Encyclopedia *Ascorbic acid*
...accelerating the emergence of human beings: Challem, J., & Taylor, E. (1998). Retroviruses, Ascorbate, and Mutations, in the

Evolution of Homo sapiens. *Free Radical Biology and Medicine,* *25*(1), 130-132.

However, there was considerable variance between specific primate species: Hooker, J. (1992). 25. British Mammalian Paleocommunities across the Eocene-Oligocene Transition and Their Environmental Implications. *Eocene-Oligocene Climatic and Biotic Evolution.*

Possible elements of this experimentation might include the following: There are many sources distilled here, the main one being http://adventure.howstuffworks.com/universal-edibility-test.htm, accessed May, 2015.

...howler monkey, in which it is found that they do not satiate with a found preferred food source but will mix into their diet other fruits and leafy plants: Milton, K. (1993). Diet and Primate Evolution. *Scientific American*, 86-93.

...to avoid over-consumption from a single plant species with, for example, a toxic component: Strier, K. (2000). *Primate behavioral ecology.* Boston: Allyn and Bacon.

20 MYA to 7 MYA

...they were not well suited for breaking down tough plant foods such as stems and soft seed pods: Simopoulos, A., & Eaton et al., S. (1998). Dietary intake of long-chain polyunsaturated fatty acids during the Paleolithic. In *The return of w3 fatty acids into the food supply: International Conference on the Return of w3 Fatty Acids into the Food Supply, I. Land-Based Animal Food Products, Bethesda, Md., September 18-19, 1997* (pp. 12-23). Basel, CH: Karger.

These were the last common ancestors (LCA) of both humans and the modern ape family: Groves, C., & Burenhult, G. (1993). *Our Earliest Ancestors. In The First Humans: Human Origins and History to 10,000 B.C.* (pp. 42-43). New York: Harper-Collins.

...chimps and gorillas qualitatively seem to be more related to each other than chimps to humans: Lieberman, D. (2013). *The story of the human body: Evolution, health, and disease* (Kindle ed., pp. 488-493). Knopf Doubleday Publishing Group.

7 MYA to 4.5 MYA

This time interval saw the emergence of the first known hominid (proto-human) known as the *root ape: Ardipithecus ramidus.*

This earliest of hominid was at least a part-time biped that subsisted on a fairly generalized plant-based diet to have included fruit, leaves, and probably some nuts, seeds, and roots: Tattersall, I. (2012). Masters of the planet: The search for our human origins (p. 8). St. Martin's Press.

4.5 MYA to 2.5 MYA

Moreover, changes in diet-related adaptations suggest that hard, abrasive foods such as seeds, nuts, and roots became increasingly important through this period, perhaps even as critical items in the diet: Teaford, M., & Ungar, P. (2000). Diet and the evolution of the earliest human ancestors. *Proceedings of the National Academy of Sciences, 10*(1073), 13506-13511.

Bipedal specializations are found in hominid fossils from about 4.2-3.9 million years ago: McHenry, H., Ruse, M., & Travis, J. (2009). Human Evolution. In *Evolution: The First Four Billion Years*

(p. 263). Cambridge, Massachusetts: The Belknap Press of Harvard University Press.

...other dietary modifications and inclusions not of an animal derived nature, such as *underground storage organs* (USO) might have been the keystone resources for these hominids: Wrangham, R., Jones, J., Laden, G., Pilbeam, D., & Conklin-Brittain, N. (1999). The Raw and the Stolen: Cooking and the Ecology of Human Origins. *Current Anthropology, 40,* 567-594.

In fact, one might speculate that a diet rich in USOs was so effective that it partly made possible their remarkable adaptive radiation: Lieberman, D. (2013). *The story of the human body: Evolution, health, and disease.* Knopf Doubleday Publishing Group.

USOs are more starchy and energy rich than many wild fruits: Laden, G., & Wrangham, R. (2005). The rise of the hominids as an adaptive shift in fallback foods: Plant underground storage organs (USOs) and australopith origins. *Journal of Human Evolution, 49,* 482-498.

Adaptive dietary diversity

In order to illustrate the range of these dietary changes, consider the accompanying figure, a so-called *right angle mixture triangle:* Raubenheimer, D., Machovsky-Capuska, G., Chapman, C., & Rothman, J. (2014). Geometry of nutrition in field studies: An illustration using wild primates. Oecologia, 117, 223-234.

...rich in micronutrients such as copper, iron, magnesium, manganese, phosphorous, selenium, and zinc, as well as riboflavin, pantothenic acid, biotin, and other vitamins and minerals in varying quantities: Rumpold, B., & Schlüter, O. (2013). Nutritional composition and safety aspects of edible insects.

Molecular Nutrition & Food Research Mol. Nutr. Food Res., 57(5), 802-823.

This is represented on the RAM: Represents 10% caloric ratio from fat, 15% protein, 75% carbohydrates: Barnard, N., Cohen, J., Jenkins, D., Turner-Mcgrievy, G., Gloede, L., Jaster, B., . . . Talpers, S. (2006). A Low-Fat Vegan Diet Improves Glycemic Control and Cardiovascular Risk Factors in a Randomized Clinical Trial in Individuals With Type 2 Diabetes. *Diabetes Care, 29*, 1777-1783.

Chapter Three
The Paleo Times

Stone: product release 1.0

Tools of this type are classified as *Mode 1* under a scheme proposed by Sir Grahame Clark, whereby stone tools are classified into five categories or "modes" that range from the simplest (Mode 1) to most complex (Mode 5): Lewin, R., & Foley, R. (2004). *Principles of human evolution* (2nd ed.). Malden, MA: Blackwell Pub.

From about 2.5 million years ago: Tattersall, I. (2012). *Masters of the planet: The search for our human origins* (MacSci) (p. 38). St. Martin's Press.

Attribution, illustration "Chopping tool" by José-Manuel Benito Álvarez. Licensed under CC BY-SA 2.5 via Wikimedia Commons - https://commons.wikimedia.org/wiki/File:Chopping_tool.gif#/media/File:Chopping_tool.gif

Stone Version 2.0

This is Mode 2 of the Lewin and Foley classification mentioned earlier.

The next technological advance was a creative leap about 1.5 million years ago: the *hand axe*: Lepre, C., Roche, H., Kent, D., Harmand, S., Quinn, R., Brugal, J., . . . Feibel, C. (2011). An earlier origin for the Acheulian. *Nature, 477,* 82-85.

Attribution, illustration "Hand axe spanish" by José-Manuel Benito - Own work. Licensed under Public Domain via Wikimedia Commons   - https://commons.wikimedia.org/wiki/File:Hand_axe_spanish.gif# /media/File:Hand_axe_spanish.gif

Out of Africa

A later migration of far more intelligent progeny more than a million years later established advanced hominids over all land masses on the planet: Lewin, R. (1997). Distant Cousins. *New Scientist,* 5-5.

How often were these opportunistic scavenging events? Difficult to say but likely infrequent: Lupo, K and J. O'Connell, (Jan 2002) Cut and Tooth Mark Distributions on Large Animal Bones: Ethnoarchaeological Data from the Hadza and Their Implications For Current Ideas About Early Human Carnivory, J Archaeological Sci 29 (1), 85.

Advanced stone age products

This takes us to about 250,000 years ago or the last *ten per cent* of the Paleo Age: Seddon, C. (2014). *Humans: From the beginning: From the first apes to the first cities.*

True stone projectile weapons did not appear until after 40,000 years ago, or about the last 1.6% of the Paleo Age. Shea, J. (2006). The origins of lithic projectile point technology: Evidence from Africa, the Levant, and Europe. *Journal of Archaeological Science, 33*(6), 823-846.

Mitochondrial Eve

Tierney, J. (1988). The Search for Adam and Eve. *Newsweek, 111,* 46-52.

Man fire food

At a place called Qesem Cave, *modern man* apparently gathered around a fire reusing the same spot many times by about 200,000 years ago: Karkanas, P., Shahackgross, R., Ayalon, A., Barmatthews, M., Barkai, R., Frumkin, A., . . . Stiner, M. (2007). Evidence for habitual use of fire at the end of the Lower Paleolithic: Site-formation processes at Qesem Cave, Israel. *Journal of Human Evolution, 53,* 197-212.

...an area for burning wood and an adjacent cooking surface that indicate the emergence of cooking around this time: Pennisi, E. (1999). Did Cooked Tubers Spur the Evolution of Big Brains? *Science, 283*(5410), 2004-2005.

...cooked tubers alone played a more important role than cooked meat in our ancestral dietary transitions: Wrangham, R., Jones, J.,

Laden, G., Pilbeam, D., & Conklin-Brittain, N. (1999). The Raw and the Stolen: Cooking and the Ecology of Human Origins. *Current Anthropology, 40*(5), 567-594.

...for males to demonstrate their skill and fitness-related qualities as a potential mate or ally to the rest of the community: Fullager, R. (2003). Hunter, Scavenger, Grandmother, Yam. *Nature Australia, 27*(11).

...chimpanzee hunting yields more social than nutritional benefits: Dunbar, R. (1988). *Primate social systems.* Ithaca, N.Y.: Comstock Pub. Associates, Cornell University Press.

...given that time and expended energy is an important additional constraint on energy intake: Dunbar, R. (1988). *Primate social systems.* Ithaca, N.Y.: Comstock Pub. Associates, Cornell University Press.

For example, female chimpanzees are more likely to have sex with males who have shared meat with them than with those that have not: Gomes, C., & Boesch, C. (2009). Wild Chimpanzees Exchange Meat for Sex on a Long-Term Basis. *PLoS ONE, 4*(5116).

...yams, which would have been super abundant on the African landscape for millions of years: Fullagar, Richard, (Summer2003/2004) Hunter, scavenger, grandmother, yam.

Autoimmune disease and meat

N-Glycolylneuraminic acid: Michael Greger MD has a series of videos on this topic on his fact-filled website nutritionfacts.org; search "Neu5Gc."

Thus Neu5Gc was introduced into the human diet, a *tumor promoter:* Hedlund, M., Padler-Karavani, V., Varki, N., & Varki, A.

(2008). Evidence for a human-specific mechanism for diet and antibody-mediated inflammation in carcinoma progression. *Proceedings of the National Academy of Sciences, 105*(48), 18936-18941.

Recall also that the ability of primates to self-manufacture the carbohydrate alpha-gal: Galactose-alpha-1,3-galactose

The anti-alpha-gal antibody is involved in a number of detrimental process that may result in allergic, autoimmune, and autoimmune-like pathogeneses: Galili, U. (2013). Anti-Gal: An abundant human natural antibody of multiple pathogeneses and clinical benefits. *Immunology, 140*(1), 1-11.

Dietary patterns in the Paleolithic Age

The preponderance of evidence supports the assertion that plant foods were predominant in the diets of hunter-gatherers: Mitton K (2000) Hunter-gatherer diets – a different perspective. *American Journal of Clinical Nutrition* **71**: 665–7.

Chapter Four
The Purpose Driven Plant

!Kung informant: Quoted by Richard Lee in "What hunters do for a living, or how to make out on scarce resources", Lee, R., & Devore, I. (1968). What hunters do for a living, or how to make out on scarce resources. In *Man the hunter*. New York: Aldine de Gruyter.

Agriculture originated independently in several parts of the world: Ulijaszek, S., & Mann, N. (2012). Evolving human nutrition:

Implications for public health (Kindle ed., pp. 351-353). New York: Cambridge University Press.

The founder crops were einkorn and emmer wheat, barley, lentils, peas, flax, bitter vetch, chickpea, and possibly fava beans: Brown, T., Jones, M., Powell, W., & Allaby, R. (2009). The complex origins of domesticated crops in the Fertile Crescent. *Trends in Ecology & Evolution, 24*, 103-109.

Emergence of grains and legumes

When the grains came

One such grouping, Ohalo II: Weiss E, Kislev ME, Simchoni O, Nadel D, Tschauner H (2008) Plant-food preparation area on an Upper Paleolithic brush hut floor at Ohalo II, Israel. *J Archaeol Sci* **35**:2400–2414.

Evidence of starch grains from various wild plants was found on the surfaces of grinding tools at the sites of Bilancino II (Italy), Kostenki 16 (Russia), and Pavlov VI (Czech Republic): Revedin A, Aranguren B, Svoboda J, et al. (2010), Thirty thousand-year-old evidence of plant food processing. Proceedings of The National Academy of Sciences of The United States of America 107(44),18815-18819.

Recent excavations in the Kebara Cave in Israel revealed charred remains of 3313 seeds, 78.8% belonging to the legume family: Lev E, Kislev M, Bar-Yosef O. Mousterian vegetal food in Kebara Cave, Mt. Carmel. *Journal Of Archaeological Science* [serial online]. March 2005;32(3):475-484.

...including those of sorghum grasses: Mercader, J. (2009), Mozambican Grass Seed Consumption During the Middle Stone Age, Science, 326.

Domestication of animals

...cattle following at about 8000 years ago: Dobney, K., & Larson, G. (2006). Genetics and animal domestication: New windows on an elusive process. *Journal of Zoology, 269*, 261-271.

Vascular disease

Data from various lines of evidence – anatomic, physiologic, and paleontologic – support the view that the ancestral line of humans was strongly herbivorous; certainly animal flesh was absent: K Milton (2000). Back to basics: why foods of wild primates have relevance for modern human health. *Nutrition*, 16(7-8), 480-3.

Therefore, we evolved mechanisms not only to synthesize necessary cholesterol but to hold on to it tightly: D J Jenkins, C W Kendall, A Marchie, A L Jenkins, P W Connelly, P J Jones, V Vuksan (2003). The Garden of Eden--plant based diets, the genetic drive to conserve cholesterol and its implications for heart disease in the 21st century. *Comp Biochem Physiol A Mol Integr Physiol*, 136(1), 141-51.

This is in marked contrast to carnivores: they evolved to eat animal flesh and cannot develop vascular disease from its consumption: W C Roberts (1990), We think we are one, we act as if we are one, but we are not one. Am J Cardiol, 66(10), 896.

Genetic mutations

Research reveals intolerance is more common globally than lactase persistence (about 75% intolerant), and that the variation is genetic: Pribila, B., Hertzler, S., Martin, B., Weaver, C., & Savaiano, D. (2000). Improved Lactose Digestion and Intolerance

Among African-American Adolescent Girls Fed a Dairy Rich-Diet. *Journal of the American Dietetic Association, 100*(5), 524-528.

Based on living populations, estimates for the time of appearance of this lactase persistence mutation are within the last 10,000 to 5,000 years: Bersaglieri, T., Sabeti, P., Patterson, N., Vanderploeg, T., Schaffner, S., Drake, J., . . . Hirschhorn, J. (2004). Genetic Signatures of Strong Recent Positive Selection at the Lactase Gene. *The American Journal of Human Genetics, 74,* 1111-1120.

...has accelerated in the past 1,000 to 3,000 years, a very recent incomplete genetic modification: Allentoft, M.E., (11 June 2015), Population Genomics of Bronze Age Eurasia, *Nature* 522, 167–172.

...enzyme in farming populations has increased: Patin, E. and Quintana-Murci, L. (2008), Demeter's legacy: rapid changes to our genome imposed by diet, 23(2), 56-59.

...the emergence of this increased frequency of the protective form of ApoE can be traced to within the past 200,000 years: Fullerton, S., Clark, A., Weiss, K., Nickerson, D., Taylor, S., Stengård, J., . . . Sing, C. (2000). Apolipoprotein E Variation at the Sequence Haplotype Level: Implications for the Origin and Maintenance of a Major Human Polymorphism. *The American Journal of Human Genetics, 67*(4), 881-900.

...resulting in a crowding of the teeth: Pickrell, J. (2005, February 19). Human 'dental chaos' linked to evolution of cooking. Retrieved October 7, 2011, from http://www.newscientist.com/article/dn7035-human-dental-chaos-linked-to-evolution-of-cooking.html#.VXPcwppViko certainly past the estimated life expectancy of that era of 25 years: M Nestle(2000), Paleolithic diets: a skeptical view. Nutrition Bulletin 25 (1), 43-47.

In short, there is no genetic evidence that we have evolved to favor the consumption of animal products: Harris M & Ross EB *et al.* (1987), *Food and Evolution: Toward a Theory of Human Food Habits.* Temple University Press, Philadelphia, PA.

Infectious diseases

...and pertussis (whooping cough) from pigs and dogs: Diamond, J. (1992). *The third chimpanzee: The evolution and future of the human animal.* New York, NY: HarperCollins.

Not until more recent times did average height begin to increase, but it has still not reached hunter-gatherer levels: Diamond, J. (1997). *Guns, germs, and steel: The fates of human societies.* London: Chatto and Windus.

Domestication of plants

In South America, the potato and peanuts were early domesticated crops: Piperno, D., Ranere, A., Holst, I., Iriarte, J., & Dickau, R. (2009). Starch grain and phytolith evidence for early ninth millennium B.P. maize from the Central Balsas River Valley, Mexico. *Proceedings of the National Academy of Sciences, 106*(13), 5019-5024.

Pesticidal ideations

Recently, pesticide use has been linked to neurologic disease: Kamel, F., & Hoppin, J. (2004). Association of Pesticide Exposure with Neurologic Dysfunction and Disease. *Environmental Health Perspectives, 112*(9), 950-958.

...and depression: Beard, J., Umbach, D., Hoppin, J., Richards, M., Alavanja, M., Blair, A., . . . Kamel, F. (2014). Pesticide Exposure and Depression among Male Private Pesticide Applicators in the Agricultural Health Study. *Environmental Health Perspectives, 122*(9).

Candy corn

Much of the factual material of this section is from Robinson, J. (2013, May 25). Breeding the Nutrition Out of Our Food. *New York Times.*

...plant geneticists such as Melaku Worede: Siebert, C. (2011, July 1). Food Ark. *National Geographic Magazine.*

Experts estimate that we have lost more than half of the world's food varieties over the past century: Siebert, C. (2011, July 1). Food Ark. *National Geographic Magazine.*

Chemical plants

Auxin

Other substances have value to the plant but no known value to animals; for example growth regulators like auxin: Lee, R., & Cho, H. (2013). Auxin, the organizer of the hormonal/ environmental signals for root hair growth. *Frontiers in Plant Science.*

Ethylene

Ethylene is produced from essentially all parts of higher plants, including leaves, stems, roots, flowers, fruits, tubers, and seeds: Lin, Z., Zhong, S., & Grierson, D. (2009). Recent advances in ethylene research. *Journal of Experimental Botany, 60*(12), 3311-3336.

...kudu, a gazelle of the South African savannah: Halle, F. (1999). *In Praise of Plants* (p. 157). Portland: Timber Press.

It has been known for centuries that certain ripe fruit can signal other fruit to accelerate the ripening process: Neljubov D. (1901). "Uber die horizontale Nutation der Stengel von Pisum sativum und einiger anderen Pflanzen". Beih Bot Zentralbl 10: 128–139.

Apples and bananas emit particularly high concentrations of ethylene gas, so airtight storage of other fruit with them assists ripening: Some fruits will never ripen after being picked. This is true of most citrus, berries, grapes, pineapple, and watermelon. Not all ripening fruit of the vine becomes sweeter; ones that do include apples, pears, mangoes, and kiwis. Interestingly avocados only ripen off the vine. Jeffrey Steingarten, J. (1998). *The Man Who Ate Everything*. Vintage Books.

Industrial ethylene production – hundreds of millions of tons of it per year: Production: Growth is the Norm. (2006). *Chemical and Engineering News, 84*(28), 59-59.

Nutraceutics

Throughout history and currently, plants provide the majority of treatments for disease and suffering of human beings: Wilson, E., & Farnsworth, N. (1988). *Biodiversity* (pp. 83-97). Washington, D.C.: National Academy Press.

In the United States, at least half of the pharmaceutics approved for use in the past 30 years by the FDA are derived from plants: Veeresham, C. (2012). Natural products derived from plants as a source of drugs. *Journal of Advanced Pharmaceutical Technology & Research J Adv Pharm Tech Res*, 3(4), 200-201.

The pharmaceutical industry in the world trades about $300 billion annually: Pharmaceutical Industry. (n.d.). Retrieved from http://www.who.int/trade/glossary/story073/en/

Garlic

Greece as perhaps one of the earliest "performance enhancing" agents: Green, O., & Polydoris, N. (1993). *Garlic, cancer and heart disease: Review and recommendations* (pp. 21-41). Chicago, Ill.: GN Communications (Pub.).

Because garlic was one of the earliest documented examples of plants employed for treatment of disease and maintenance of health: Kahn, G., & Lawson, L. (1996). History of Garlic. In *Garlic: The Science and Therapeutic Application of Allium sativum L. and Related Species* (pp. 25-36). New York, NY: Williams and Wilkins. Much of the information in the subsection *Garlic* was obtained from this source.

The earliest known references: Moyers, S. (1996). *Garlic in health, history, and world cuisine* (pp. 1-36). St. Petersburg, FL: Suncoast Press.

The authoritative medical text of the era was the *Codex Ebers:* Bergner, P. (1996). *The healing power of garlic* (pp. 3-26). Rocklin, Calif.: Prima Pub.

...may be most adept at blocking human cancer cell growth: Boivin, D., Lamy, S., Lord-Dufour, S., Jackson, J., Beaulieu, E., Côté,

M., . . . Béliveau, R. (2009). Antiproliferative and antioxidant activities of common vegetables: A comparative study. *Food Chemistry, 112*(2), 374-380.

She came to the conclusion that raw garlic had more health benefits than cooked garlic, a point of view verified more recently: However if raw crushed garlic is allowed to sit ten minutes or so, enzymatically assisted chemical reactions fixate healthy compounds that are resistant to heat.

The therapeutic efficacy of garlic does in fact encompass a wide variety of ailments, including cardiovascular, cancer, hepatic and microbial infections, to name but a few: Banerjee, S., Mukherjee, P., & Maulik, S. (2003). Garlic as an antioxidant: The good, the bad and the ugly. *Phytotherapy Research Phytother. Res., 17*(2), 97-106.

Food as medicine before written history

The leaves encourage clotting: Moore, M. (1997). Specific Indications in Clinical Practice. Retrieved May 19, 2013.

...and reduce pain: Noureddini, M., & Rasta, V. (2008). Analgesic Effect of aqueous extract of Achillea millefolium L. on rat's formalin test. *Pharmacology Online, 3,* 659-664.

Psychiatry's founding fodder

It was not until 1931 that five alkaloids were isolated from the plant, of the phenothiazine family: Alexander, F., & Selesnick, S. (1966). *The history of psychiatry; an evaluation of psychiatric thought and practice from prehistoric times to the present,* (p. 288). New York: Harper & Row.

Laborit did not find the effect that he sought but did note a curious *désintéressement* (disinterest) present in the patients receiving the drug: Shorter, E. (1997). *A history of psychiatry: From the era of the asylum to the age of Prozac* (pp. 249-250). New York: John Wiley & Sons.

Take two

...in 1900 as Aspirin (acetylsalicylic acid) by Bayer: Interestingly, Aspirin ® and Heroin ® were once trademarks belonging to Bayer. After Germany lost World War I, Bayer was forced to give up both trademarks as part of the Treaty of Versailles in 1919.

About one in ten people on chronic low-dose aspirin develop stomach or intestinal ulcers, which can perforate the gut and cause life-threatening bleeding: Yeomans, N., Lanas, A., Talley, N., Thomson, A., Daneshjoo, R., Eriksson, B., . . . Hawkey, C. (2005). Prevalence and incidence of gastroduodenal ulcers during treatment with vascular protective doses of aspirin. *Aliment Pharmacol Ther Alimentary Pharmacology and Therapeutics, 22*(9), 795-801.

All plants contain salicylic acid and vegetarians have as much in their blood as omnivores who take aspirin supplements - but without the risk: Paterson, J., Baxter, G., Dreyer, J., Halket, J., Flynn, R., & Lawrence, J. (2008). Salicylic Acid sans Aspirin in Animals and Man: Persistence in Fasting and Biosynthesis from Benzoic Acid. *Journal of Agricultural and Food Chemistry J. Agric. Food Chem., 56*(24), 11648-11652.

...the immune system of plants by activating the production of pathogen-fighting proteins: Pieterse, C., Van Der Does, C., Zamioudis, C., Leon-Reyes, A., & Van Wees, S. (2012). *Hormonal modulation of plant immunity.* Annu Rev Cell Dev Biol.

It can transmit the distress signal throughout the plant and even to neighboring plants: Taiz, L., & Zeiger, E. (2002). *Plant physiology* (3rd ed., p. 306). New York: W.H. Freeman.

Recently, mental disorders have been linked to chronic inflammatory states: Berk, M., Dean, O., Drexhage, H., McNeil, J. J., Moylan, S., O'Neil, A., ... Maes, M. (2013). Aspirin: a review of its neurobiological properties and therapeutic potential for mental illness. *BMC Medicine, 11*, 74. doi:10.1186/1741-7015-11-74.

...aspirin is finding a use for disorders ranging from mood disorders: Ayorech, Z., Tracy, D., Baumeister, D., & Giaroli, G. (2015). Taking the fuel out of the fire: Evidence for the use of anti-inflammatory agents in the treatment of bipolar disorders. *Journal of Affective Disorders, 174*, 467-478.

...to schizophrenia: Keller, W., Kum, L., Wehring, H., Koola, M., Buchanan, R., & Kelly, D. (2012). A review of anti-inflammatory agents for symptoms of schizophrenia. *Journal of Psychopharmacology (Oxford, England), 27*(4), 337-342.

Chapter Five
The Science, Art, and Psychology of Eating

There are many potential invaders, so plants produce an enormous number of compounds that are toxic, repellent, or antinutritive for herbivores of all types: Mithöfer, A., & Boland, W. (2012). Plant Defense Against Herbivores: Chemical Aspects. *Annu. Rev. Plant Biol. Annual Review of Plant Biology, 63*, 431-450.

Let's explore several types of phytonutrients including anti-inflammatories, antioxidants, and fiber: A great deal of information on each of these topics may be researched in an entertaining video format on Dr. Michael Greger's website nutritionfacts.org.

These secondary metabolites of plants, numbering in the hundreds of thousands: Campbell, T. C. (2013, March). Lecture on Food Science. *Holistic Holiday at Sea.*

We just don't know yet: "Consuming anti-microbial compounds (as well as other compounds) synthesized by plants as part of their immune response may be beneficial to human immunity. That is the only connection that I see between plant and human immunity", Ausubel, Frederick M, Department of Genetics, Harvard Medical School, Boston, Massachusetts private communication, July 2012.

Epidemiological data as well as human intervention studies suggest that dietary patterns that emphasize fruit and vegetables are strongly inversely proportional to affect inflammatory processes: Watzl, B. (2008). Anti-inflammatory Effects of Plant-based Foods and of their Constituents. *International Journal for Vitamin and Nutrition Research, 78*(6), 293-298.

They serve two key roles in plants: they absorb light energy for use in photosynthesis, and they protect chlorophyll from photodamage: Armstrong, G., & Hearst, J. (1996). Carotenoids 2: Genetics and molecular biology of carotenoid pigment biosynthesis. *FASEB J, 10*(2), 228-237.

Flavonoids are also present in a wide variety of plants: Spencer, J. (2008). Flavonoids: Modulators of brain function? *BJN British Journal of Nutrition, 99,* 60-77.

We know that a single meal high in animal fat can cause an elevation in inflammation within our bodies that peaks at about four hours: Vogel, R., Corretti, M., & Plotnick, G. (1997). Effect of a

153

Single High-Fat Meal on Endothelial Function in Healthy Subjects. *The American Journal of Cardiology, 79*(3), 350-354.

We know that a single meal high in animal fat can cause an elevation in inflammation within our bodies that peaks at about four hours: Vogel, R., Corretti, M., & Plotnick, G. (1997). Effect of a Single High-Fat Meal on Endothelial Function in Healthy Subjects. *The American Journal of Cardiology, 79*(3), 350-354.

Bacteria: The unseen majority

Gut check

It is the bacteria present in *meat products and processed foods* that bring the endotoxins: Erridge, C. (2010). The capacity of foodstuffs to induce innate immune activation of human monocytes in vitro is dependent on food content of stimulants of Toll-like receptors 2 and 4. *Br J Nutr British Journal of Nutrition, 105*(1), 15-23.

The B$_{12}$ issue

The soil bacteria called *Rhizobia* that fixes nitrogen after being taken in by plant root nodules make it: Herbert, V. (1988). Vitamin B-12: Plant sources, requirements, and assay. *The American Journal of Clinical Nutrition, 48*(3), 852-858.

Taming the fire – the purpose of antioxidants

This need for antioxidants is even greater during photosynthesis, where very highly reactive oxygen intermediates are produced: Demmig-Adams, B. (2002). Antioxidants in Photosynthesis and Human Nutrition. *Science, 298*(5601), 2149-2153.

As plants adapted to a terrestrial environment from marine life, they began producing non-marine antioxidants such as ascorbic acid: Padayatty, S., Katz, A., Wang, Y., Eck, P., Kwon, O., Lee, J., . . . Levine, M. (2003). Vitamin C as an Antioxidant: Evaluation of Its Role in Disease Prevention. *Journal of the American College of Nutrition, 22*(1), 18-35.

...compounds that reflect certain wavelengths of sunlight, appearing as various colors: Benzie, J. (2003). Evolution of dietary antioxidants. *Comparative Biochemistry and Physiology, 136*(1), 113-126.

Although the human body has developed a number of systems to eliminate free radicals, such as reactive oxygen species from the body, it is not very efficient: Seeram, N., Aviram, M., Zhang, Y., Henning, S., Feng, L., Dreher, M., & Heber, D. (2008). Comparison of Antioxidant Potency of Commonly Consumed Polyphenol-Rich Beverages in the United States. *Journal of Agricultural and Food Chemistry J. Agric. Food Chem., 56,* 1415-1422.

Without sufficient intake of protective antioxidants, only found in plants, excessive intake of the typical energy-dense foods of Western societies can result in cellular dysfunction, disease, and death: Prior, R., Gu, L., Wu, X., Jacob, R., Sotoudeh, G., Kader, A., & Cook, R. (2007). Plasma Antioxidant Capacity Changes Following a Meal as a Measure of the Ability of a Food to Alter In Vivo Antioxidant Status. *Journal of the American College of Nutrition, 26*(2), 170-181.

The China Study: Campbell, T., & Campbell, T. (2005). The China study: The most comprehensive study of nutrition ever conducted and the startling implications for diet, weight loss and long-term health. Dallas, Tex.: BenBella Books.

Whole: Rethinking the Science of Nutrition: Campbell, T., & Jacobson, H. (2014). *Whole: Rethinking the Science of Nutrition.* BenBella Books.

In effect, the 'whole' nutritional effect is greater than the sum of its parts: The Daily Beet. (n.d.). Retrieved May 27, 2015, from http://engine2diet.com/the-daily-beet/the-big-oil-post-plus-a-giveaway

Food synergy

Less than one half of one percent of all money for medical research is spent on nutrition largely because there are no patented, profitable drugs that result: The Influence of Nutrition on Mental Health (Part 2) - Charis Holistic Center. (2011, October 26). Retrieved May 27, 2015, from http://www.charisholisticcenter.com/the-influence-of-nutrition-on-mental-health-part-2/

Most research conducted takes the reductionist approach aimed at identifying the molecules involved in biological events and examining them in their purified form or in simple systems: Zeisel, S., Allen, L., Coburn, S., Erdman, J., Failla, M., Freake, H., . . . Storch, J. (2001). Nutrition: A reservoir of integrative science. *J Nutr, 131,* 1319–1321-1319–1321.

For example, the plant turmeric, containing the ingredient curcumin, appears to have a wide range of biological effects including anti-inflammatory, antioxidant, antibacterial, and antiviral: Aggarwal, B., Sundaram, C., Malani, N., & Ichikawa, H. (2007). Curcumin: The Indian Solid Gold. *The Molecular Targets and Therapeutic Uses of Curcumin in Health and Disease Advances in Experimental Medicine and Biology, 595*(1), 1-75.

Extracts of phytonutrients, such as curcumin just mentioned, could have deleterious effects: Cao, J., Jia, L., & Zhong, L. (2006). Mitochondrial and Nuclear DNA Damage Induced by Curcumin in Human Hepatoma G2 Cells. *Toxicological Sciences, 91*(2), 476-483.

Tomatoes and broccoli both have anti-prostate tumor properties but the combination is better than the sum of the effects individually: The reason for this enhancement is unknown; Canene-Adams, K., Lindshield, B., Wang, S., Jeffery, E., Clinton, S., & Erdman, J. (2007). Combinations of Tomato and Broccoli Enhance Antitumor Activity in Dunning R3327-H Prostate Adenocarcinomas. *Cancer Research, 67,* 836-843.

Eating two different fruits together has a greater antioxidant capacity than the same amount of either fruit consumed individually: Liu, R. (2003). Health benefits of fruit and vegetables are from additive and synergistic combinations of phytochemicals. *The American Journal of Clinical Nutrition, 78*(3), 517S-520S.

Vitamin C helps to make iron more absorbable so a combination of fruit with iron containing vegetables (leeks, beet greens, kale, spinach, etc.) may be particularly effective for this purpose: Weber, J., & Zimmerman, M. (2009). *The men's health big book of food & nutrition: Your completely delicious guide to eating well, looking great, and staying lean for life!* (p. 102). New York: Rodale.

More bang for the bulk

Even the definition of *fiber* is not consistently accepted: Consider those of the Institute of Medicine (Institute of Medicine; Food and Nutrition Board. Dietary Reference Intakes: energy, carbohydrates, fiber, fat, fatty acids, cholesterol, protein and amino acids. Washington (DC): National Academies Press; 2005.) and that of the Codex Alimentarius Commission (Codex Alimentarius Commission; Food and Agriculture Organization;

World Health Organization. Report of the 30th session of the Codex Committee on nutrition and foods for special dietary uses. ALINORM 9/32/26. 2009).

Furthermore, there may be digestible important phytonutrients that are chemically attached to the fibrous content and released during processing by our micro flora: Arranz, S., Silván, J., & Saura-Calixto, F. (2010). Nonextractable polyphenols, usually ignored, are the major part of dietary polyphenols: A study on the Spanish diet. *Molecular Nutrition & Food Research Mol. Nutr. Food Res., 54*(11), 1646-1658.

Food as art

A sentiment of some individuals in advanced societies is *the earth without art* is *"eh"*: If this is not obvious, subtract the letters art from the word earth leading to the remaining letters *eh* a colloquialism for blandness.

Neurogastronomy

Much of this section is based on facts presented by Shepherd, G. (2013). *Neurogastronomy: How the brain creates flavor and why it matters* (Reprint ed.). New York: Columbia University Press.

However *flavor*, being an interpretive higher cognitive function, can be influenced by association: We shall use the word *taste* as a noun to mean the sensations of the sweet, sour, bitter, or salty quality of a food. Taste or tasting as a verb will be taken to mean to sense the flavor of a food.

This is represented in the accompanying figure using the acronym TATER, where the letters stand for: T = Trigger; AT = automatic thought; E = emotion; and R = response: Aiken, Richard, "The Cognitive Milieu", manuscript in preparation, 2015.

Furthermore, CBT principles can be used to develop and adhere to a healthy dietary pattern as it becomes part of one's natural lifestyle: Beck, J. (2009). *The Beck diet solution: Train your brain to think like a thin person* (Reprint ed.). Birmingham, Ala.: Oxmoor House.

Fork in the road

Within the evolutionary medicine literature, the origin of agriculture tends to be seen as the primary point at which dietary 'adaptation' switches to 'maladaptation' within humans: Simopoulos, A., & Eaton et al., S. (1998). Dietary intake of long-chain polyunsaturated fatty acids during the Paleolithic. In *The return of w3 fatty acids into the food supply: International Conference on the Return of w3 Fatty Acids into the Food Supply, I. Land-Based Animal Food Products, Bethesda, Md., September 18-19, 1997* (pp. 12-23). Basel, CH: Karger.

Chapter Six
Mood Food

One such study in that issue is titled "Association of Western and Traditional Diets With Depression and Anxiety in Women: Jacka, F., Pasco, J., Mykletun, A., Williams, L., Hodge, A., O'reilly, S., . . . Berk, M. (2010). Association of Western and Traditional Diets With Depression and Anxiety in Women. *AJP American Journal of Psychiatry, 167*(3), 305-311.

Another study looking at the relationship of diet to mood in adults is titled "Dietary pattern and depressive symptoms in middle age: Akbaraly, T., Brunner, E., Ferrie, J., Marmot, M., Kivimaki, M., & Singh-Manoux, A. (2009). Dietary pattern and depressive symptoms in middle age. *The British Journal of Psychiatry, 195*(5), 408-413. doi:10.1192/bjp.bp.108.058925.

Another large and recent prospective cohort study performed at the University College London: Akbaraly, T., Sabia, S., Shipley, M., Batty, G., & Kivimaki, M. (2013). Adherence to healthy dietary guidelines and future depressive symptoms: Evidence for sex differentials in the Whitehall II study. *American Journal of Clinical Nutrition,* 97(2), 419-427.

There are a number of other studies that make similar claims of improving mood in adults with better dietary patterns, such as a study performed at the University of Delaware reported in 2010: Kuczmarski, M., Sees, A., Hotchkiss, L., Cotugna, N., Evans, M., & Zonderman, A. (2010). Higher Healthy Eating Index-2005 Scores Associated with Reduced Symptoms of Depression in an Urban Population: Findings from the Healthy Aging in Neighborhoods of Diversity Across the Life Span (HANDLS) Study. *Journal of the American Dietetic Association, 110*(3), 383-389.

And another at the University of Calgary in 2012: Davison, K., & Kaplan, B. (2012). Nutrient intakes are correlated with overall psychiatric functioning in adults with mood disorders. *Canadian Journal of Psychiatry. Revue Canadienne De Psychiatrie, 57*(2), 85-92.

One such study of the Mediterranean Diet, published in 2009 by a group at a Spanish University: Sánchez-Villegas, A., Delgado-Rodríguez, M., Alonso, A., Schlatter, J., Lahortiga, F., Majem, L., & Martínez-González, M. (2009). Association of the Mediterranean Dietary Pattern With the Incidence of Depression. *Arch Gen Psychiatry Archives of General Psychiatry, 66*(10), 1090-1098.

160

Another large prospective cohort epidemiologic investigation was reported recently by researchers at Loma Linda University: Ford, P., Jaceldo-Siegl, K., Lee, J., Youngberg, W., & Tonstad, S. (2013). Intake of Mediterranean foods associated with positive affect and low negative affect. *Journal of Psychosomatic Research, 74*(2), 142-148.

...the major dietary source of *eicosapentaenoic acid* and *docosahexaenoic acid*, critical regulators of brain cell structure and function: Beezhold, B., Johnston, C., & Daigle, D. (2010). Vegetarian diets are associated with healthy mood states: A cross-sectional study in Seventh Day Adventist adults. *Nutr J Nutrition Journal, 9*, 26-26.

...patients were randomly selected to receive three different diets over a two week time interval: Beezhold, B., & Johnston, C. (2012). Restriction of meat, fish, and poultry in omnivores improves mood: A pilot randomized controlled trial. *Nutr J Nutrition Journal, 11*, 9-9.

Teen dietary patterns – junk food, junk moods

Significant increases in the prevalence of adolescent emotional distress and behavioral problems have occurred over the past several generations: Twenge, J., Gentile, B., Dewall, C., Ma, D., Lacefield, K., & Schurtz, D. (2010). Birth cohort increases in psychopathology among young Americans, 1938–2007: A cross-temporal meta-analysis of the MMPI. *Clinical Psychology Review, 30*, 145-154.

...decreasing consumption of raw fruits, high-nutrient vegetables and associated increases in fast food, snacks and sweetened beverages: Cavadini, C. (2000). US adolescent food intake trends from 1965 to 1996. *Western Journal of Medicine, 173*, 378-383.

...with resulting obesity: Ogden, C. (2002). Prevalence and Trends in Overweight Among US Children and Adolescents, 1999-2000. *JAMA, 288,* 1728-1732.

Poorer emotional states and behavior were seen in adolescents with a typical Western dietary pattern high in red and processed meats, takeaway foods, confectionary and refined foods compared to those who consumed more fresh fruit and vegetables: Oddy, W., Robinson, M., Ambrosini, G., O'sullivan, T., Klerk, N., Beilin, L., . . . Stanley, F. (2009). The association between dietary patterns and mental health in early adolescence. *Preventive Medicine, 49,* 39-44; see also Jacka, F., Kremer, P., Leslie, E., Berk, M., Patton, G., Toumbourou, J., & Williams, J. (2010).

Associations between diet quality and depressed mood in adolescents: Results from the Australian Healthy Neighbourhoods Study. *Aust NZ J Psychiatry Australian and New Zealand Journal of Psychiatry, 44,* 435-442.

The first prospective cohort study on the effect of diet quality on mental health of adolescents was published in 2011, based on over 3000 adolescents 11- 18 years old: Jacka, F., Kremer, P., Berk, M., Silva-Sanigorski, A., Moodie, M., Leslie, E., . . . Swinburn, B. (2011). A Prospective Study of Diet Quality and Mental Health in Adolescents. *PLoS ONE, 6*(9).

...indicated early poor nutritional exposures in utero were related to risk for behavioral and emotional problems in their children: Jacka, F., Ystrom, E., Brantsaeter, A., Karevold, E., Roth, C., Haugen, M., . . . Berk, M. (2013). Maternal and Early Postnatal Nutrition and Mental Health of Offspring by Age 5 Years: A Prospective Cohort Study. *Journal of the American Academy of Child & Adolescent Psychiatry, 52*(9), 1038-1047.

...neurologic development continues after birth and extends throughout childhood and adolescence into young adulthood: Giedd, J., & Rapoport, J. (2010). Structural MRI of Pediatric Brain Development: What Have We Learned and Where Are We Going? *Neuron, 67*(5), 728-734.

...lifetime psychiatric disorders will first emerge by late adolescence or early adulthood: Kessler, R., Berglund, P., Demler, O., Jin, R., Merikangas, K., & Walters, E. (2005). Lifetime Prevalence and Age-of-Onset Distributions of DSM-IV Disorders in the National Comorbidity Survey Replication. *Arch Gen Psychiatry Archives of General Psychiatry, 62*, 593-602.

Chapter Seven
The New Ancestral Diet

Also over thousands of millennia we lost the ability to produce the following substances: The alpha gal story is an interesting one; search this phrase on Dr. Michael Greger's informative website NutritionFacts.org.

"lips to hips": I first heard this phrase written by Dr. Joel Fuhrman, who takes a similar stance to ours on the importance of nutrient density; Fuhrman, J. (2011). Eat to Live: The Amazing Nutrient-Rich Program for Fast and Sustained Weight Loss (Vol. Revised). Boston: Little, Brown and Company.

...dietary intake can directly lead to vascular disease, including heart failure and strokes: Dr. Roberts, the Editor and Chief of the American Journal of Cardiology has been advocating cholesterol as the source of vascular disease in editorals for more than a decade, such as the following reference. Roberts, W. (2010). It's the Cholesterol, Stupid! *The American Journal of Cardiology, 106*(9), 1364-1366.

Arachidonic acid is a key substrate for the synthesis of proinflammatory compounds that can adversely affect mental health via a cascade of neuroinflammation: Beezhold, B., Johnston, C., & Daigle, D. (2010). Vegetarian diets are associated with healthy mood states: A cross-sectional study in Seventh Day Adventist adults. *Nutr J Nutrition Journal, 9,* 26-26.

Caloric macronutrient distribution

The National Academy of Sciences Institute of Medicine's Food and Nutrition Board gives the following information for macronutrient composition: *Dietary reference intakes for energy, carbohydrate, fiber, fat, fatty acids, cholesterol, protein, and amino acids.* (2005). Washington, D.C.: National Academies Press.

Physicians' Committee for Responsible Medicine: Represents 10% caloric ratio from fat, 15% protein, 75% carbohydrates. Barnard, N., Cohen, J., Jenkins, D., Turner-Mcgrievy, G., Gloede, L., Jaster, B., . . . Talpers, S. (2006). A Low-Fat Vegan Diet Improves Glycemic Control and Cardiovascular Risk Factors in a Randomized Clinical Trial in Individuals With Type 2 Diabetes. *Diabetes Care, 29,* 1777-1783.

...human breast milk, a whole food complete diet composition designed by nature as most nourishing, contains only 8% of its total calories as protein: Jenness, R. (1979). The composition of human milk. *Seminars in Perinatology, 3,* 225-239.

The Okinawa traditional diet

Tending a garden also lowers stress and increases vitamin D: Buettner, D. (2008), Blue Zones: Lessons for Living Longer from the People Who've Lived the Longest, National Geographic, Reprint edition.

The National Health and Nutrition Examination Survey is the primary national data system which provides information to monitor the nutritional status of the U.S. population: Wright, J.D. and C-Y Wang (2010), Trends in Intake of Energy and Macronutrients in Adults From 1999-2000 Through 2007-2008, NCHS Data Brief, 49.

Energy density versus nutrient density

"Percent max" on the ordinate is based on pure fat as 100% energy dense; percent max for nutrient density is based on the measure used by Nutrition Data: There are many ways to measure nutrient density and no universally acceptable way. This measure used here does not include the phytonutrients so is a lower limit on nutrition. (n.d.). Retrieved May 28, 2015, from http://nutritiondata.self.com

Fiber

Wild fruits and vegetables are the original low-glycemic foods: Robinson, J. (2013). *Eating on the wild side: The missing link to optimum health* (pp. 4-5).

It is estimated that 97% of Americans do not consume the recommended minimum amount of fiber: Moshfegh, A., & Goldman, J. (2005). What We Eat in America, NHANES 2001-2002: Usual Nutrient Intakes from Food Compared to Dietary Reference

Intakes. *U.S. Department of Agriculture, Agricultural Research Service.*

Omega-3 fatty acids

An *adequate intake*: *Adequate Intake for individual nutrients* is similar to *Recommended Dietary Allowances* but less certain.

ALA is 1.6 grams/day for men and 1.1 grams/day for women: Food and Nutrition Board. (2005). *Dietary reference intakes for energy, carbohydrate, fiber, fat, fatty acids, cholesterol, protein, and amino acids* (p. 423). Washington, D.C.: National Academies Press.

In addition, current research demonstrates that taking fish oil supplements does not actually produce significant protection on cardiovascular health: Kwak, S., Myung, S., & Lee, Y. (2012). Efficacy of omega-3 fatty acid supplements (eicosapentaenoic acid and docosahexaenoic acid) in the secondary prevention of cardiovascular disease: A meta-analysis of randomized, double-blind, placebo- controlled trials. *Archives of Internal Medicine Arch Intern Med, 172*, 986-994.

Research has shown that omega-3s are found in the more stable form, ALA, in vegetables, fruits, and beans: Odeleye, O., & Watson, R. (1991). Health implications of the n-3 fatty acids. *American Journal of Clinical Nutrition, 53*, 177-178.

...women on vegan diets actually have more EPA and DHA in their blood compared with fish-eaters, meat-eaters, and lacto-ovo vegetarians: Welch, A., Shakya-Shrestha, S., Lentjes, M., Wareham, N., & Khaw, K. (2010). Dietary intake and status of n-3 polyunsaturated fatty acids in a population of fish-eating and non-fish-eating meat-eaters, vegetarians, and vegans and the precursor-product ratio of -linolenic acid to long-chain n-3 polyunsaturated fatty acids: Results. *American Journal of Clinical Nutrition, 92*, 1040-1051.

Omega-6 to omega-3 ratio

This high ratio promotes the pathogenesis of vascular disease, cancer, and inflammatory and autoimmune diseases, whereas lower ratios exert suppressive effects: Simopoulos, A. (2002). The importance of the ratio of omega-6/omega-3 essential fatty acids. *Biomedicine & Pharmacotherapy, 56*(8), 365-379.

Wild edibles

dandelions – bet you can't eat just one

Dandelions are found worldwide: Brouillet, L. (2014). *Flora of North America North of Mexico.* New York, NY: Oxford University Press.

They are thought to have evolved about thirty million years ago: Gardening in Washington: Dandelions. (2003). from http://gardening.wsu.edu/

They are considered a noxious weed and a nuisance in residential and recreational lawns in North America: Stewart-Wade, S., Neumann, S., Collins, L., & Boland, G. (2002). The biology of Canadian weeds. 117. Taraxacum officinale G. H. Weber ex Wiggers. *Canadian Journal of Plant Science, 82*, 825-853.

piss-a-bed: Taylor, J. (1819). *Antiquitates curiosae: The etymology of many remarkable old sayings, proverbs and singular customs explained by Joseph Taylor* (2nd ed., p. 97). T&J Allman.

worm rose: "Den virtuella floran: Taraxacum F. H. Wigg. - Maskrosor" (in Swedish). Linnaeus.nrm.se

They have significant anti-inflammatory, anti-oxidative, anti-carcinogenic, analgesic, anti-hyperglycemic, anti-coagulatory, and prebiotic effects: Schütz, K., Carle, R., & Schieber, A. (2006). Taraxacum—A review on its phytochemical and pharmacological profile. *Journal of Ethnopharmacology, 107*(3), 313-323.

...higher proportions of unsaturated fatty acids (oleic, palmitoleic, linoleic, and linolenic acids): Souci, S., Fachmann, W., & Kraut, H. (2008). *Food Composition and Nutrition Tables* (7th ed.). Stuttgart: Med Pharm Scientific.

Emerging scientific evidence suggests that dandelions might have potential to prevent or ameliorate the outcome of several degenerative diseases such as atherosclerosis and coronary artery and vascular disease, obesity, diabetes mellitus, and cancer: González-Castejón, M., Visioli, F., & Rodriguez-Casado, A. (2012). Diverse biological activities of dandelion. *Nutrition Reviews, 70*(9), 534-547.

purslane

Purslane contains more omega-3 fatty acids than any other leafy vegetable plant: Omara-Alwala, T., Mebrahtu, T., Prior, D., & Ezekwe, M. (1991). Omega-three fatty acids in purslane (Portulaca oleracea) Tissues. *J Am Oil Chem Soc Journal of the American Oil Chemists' Society, 68*(3), 198-199.

...seven times more beta-carotene than carrots: Robinson, J. (2013). *Eating on the wild side: The missing link to optimum health* (p. 4).

Two types of red and yellow pigments are potent antioxidants and have been found to have antimutagenic properties in laboratory studies: Caballero-Salazar, S., Riverón-Negrete, L., Ordáz-Téllez, M., Abdullaev, F., & Espinosa-Aguirre, J. (2002). Evaluation of the antimutagenic activity of different vegetable extracts using an in vitro screening test. *Proceedings of the Western Pharmacology Society, 45,* 101-103.

stinging nettle

It contains 25% (dry weight) protein, one of the highest protein content for a leafy green vegetable: Hughes, R., Ellery, P., Harry, T., Jenkins, V., & Jones, E. (1980). The dietary potential of the common nettle. *Journal of the Science of Food and Agriculture J. Sci. Food Agric., 31*(12), 1279-1286.

Food processing

Without resorting to "pre-processing": An excellent exploration into this topic is Chef AJ and Glen Merzer's book *Unprocessed* (February, 2011).

Appendix
The epic meal

Much of what is grown we start from seeds. We use heritage seeds from Baker Creek Heirloom Seed Company: The largest online heirloom seed company in the United States and coincidently located just down the street from our ranch near Mansfield, Missouri, home of *"Little House on the Prairie"* author Laura Ingalls Wilder.

...dandelion, 12 gm: The dandelion greens are from a single plant; ironically our lawn is maintained by a service that apparently uses chemicals that discourage "weeds". This sole dandelion was found growing in a flowerpot of Missouri Primrose.

INDEX

171

O

P

Q

R

S

T

U

V

vitamin C.................... 20, 21, 72, 74, 93

Vitamix 107, 112

W

weapons 39, 134

Y

yarrow 60

Made in the USA
Lexington, KY
05 September 2018